YOU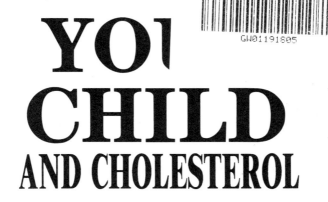
CHILD
AND CHOLESTEROL

by

Eugene Eisman, M.D. and
Diane Batshaw Eisman, M.D.

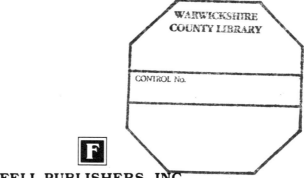

F

FELL PUBLISHERS, INC.
Hollywood, Florida

Library of Congress Cataloging-In-Publication Data

Eisman, Eugene.

Your child and cholesterol / by Eugene Eisman, M.D. and Diane Batshaw Eisman, M.D.—1st ed.
p.   cm.

ISBN 0-8119-0034-7 : $12.95
1. Children--Health and hygiene--Popular works. 2.
Children--Nutrition--Popular works.
3. Low-cholesterol diets--Recipes. 4. Exercise for
children--Popular works. I. Eisman, Diane Batshaw. II.
Title.

RJ61.E35 1991   91-83600
613'.0432--dc20   CIP

Manufactured in the United States of America
10 9 8 7 6 5 4 3 2 1

Dedication

This book is dedicated to the Batshaws and Eismans
who love food,
but not more than they enjoy good health.

Acknowledgement

The recipes have been reviewed by Chef James
Jorgenson in the interests of public safety.

CONTENTS

INTRODUCTION

Don shivered as the cold from the frozen food section hit him. Moving closer, he gazed at rows of appealing packages of fried potatoes - golden, crunchy, delicious, and so full of fat!

Fries and a hamburger — the magic combination. If you're too tired to help with homework, send the youngsters to the corner for burgers and fries, and you're still a good Dad.

He reached for some cauliflower. This is what the children should be eating. But vegetables are a tough selling job for parents! Mention the word healthy and their forks stop in mid-air.

The only green his little angels allowed on their plates was chocolate chip mint ice cream. Don returned the box, letting it nestle among the other packages of boring green things. He had to admit that he did not set a good example. He often boasted that he ate vegetables even though he really hated them. Maybe that wasn't the way to do things.

So Don went back to the cauliflower. A different package illustration caught his attention, one that didn't look like cauliflower. Breaded and fried, it even came with butter-cream sauce. But now that Don was concerned about the cholesterol his children were eating, he knew that fried vegetables swimming in butter cream sauce were not a wholesome alternative.

Don and Meg had heard a lot about cholesterol. They hadn't related it to the children until last week's PTA meeting when another couple proposed that a dietitian speak next month. That couple, the Corcorans, believed youngsters must learn to eat properly.

Meg and Don thought teenagers just naturally gobbled down milk shakes and banana splits. It was an important part of growing up and socializing. After all, they were still young; when they became adults, they could start eating salads and "good stuff". Why hunt for something extra to nag the children about? A few hours a day watching television and eating potato chips wasn't so terrible. At least they were home and out of trouble.

But Don knew he was ignoring something important: his children's lifelong well-being. It was so easy to let things stay as they were, with the youngsters a little overweight and not getting much exercise. Family food shopping was done quickly on Saturday mornings while the children stayed home eating their breakfast of lunch meat sandwiches and soft drinks. Loading the pantry with huge tins of potato chips and cookies didn't take much effort. The ingredients list on those cookies included lard, but who has time to waste reading labels?

After the meeting, he and Meg joined the Corcorans for coffee, and he watched Arnie and Beth Corcoran split a fresh fruit plate. He felt so guilty eating his apple pie a la mode he added artificial sweetener and a non-dairy substitute to his coffee. He felt even worse when Beth told him that skim milk was healthier for his heart. She said the non-dairy stuff was garbage that might actually raise his cholesterol.

After that, he and Meg did some serious talking.

This cholesterol business was important. And whatever it took, the children must understand the dangers of a high-fat diet.

Chapter I

CHOLESTEROL IN A NUTSHELL

The most common causes of death in the United States are strokes and heart attacks. These result from hardening of arteries (atherosclerosis).

The two most important risk factors for atherosclerosis are being a male and aging. On those counts there is little help. Nobody has shown that sex change operations alter our fate, and we certainly can't make the clock stand still. But there are three other major factors we can do something about: high blood pressure, cigarette smoking, and an elevated cholesterol level.

This book focuses on high cholesterol. The death rate from heart disease and stroke is directly related to the amount of cholesterol in the blood. There is no doubt that cholesterol is a killer.

Although the life-style changes we advise should be followed by everyone, the book is directed toward children. Lowering your child's cholesterol could prevent a stroke or heart attack forty or fifty years in the future. Lowering cholesterol not only prolongs life, it also improves the quality of life.

Our scientific knowledge changes at a breath-taking pace. Medicine and nutrition are no exception. What is truth today will not be truth tomorrow. By the time this book reaches the store shelves some of its information will already be considered obsolete.

In addition to the march of time and the gathering of new information, you should be aware that human nutrition is not a mathematically exact science. The data is incomplete and scientists often disagree on its interpretation. As a result not everything written here is in agreement with all members of the scientific community.

Remember also that we are discussing human beings, and we face certain limitations when it comes to experimentation upon humans. Therefore we must base many of our conclusions primarily on animal experiments and observed statistical associations. Neither technique is particularly dependable, but they are all we have. As a result, scientific studies give conflicting findings. Each must choose those he wishes to believe. We must keep our minds open and be willing to change when new-found facts demand it.

The technical side of cholesterol is left to the last chapters. From knowledge gained in the first chapters you will be able to start immediately on changes in your family's lifestyle. We cannot go on, however, without giving you a summary of the science of cholesterol.

Cholesterol is a lipid (fat) that is both manufactured in the body, and also obtained directly from food. We manufacture cholesterol from animal (including dairy) fats. Cholesterol is necessary for the manufacture of many substances vital to the body. If present in more than small amounts in the blood, it will cause hardening and narrowing of the arteries. This disease robs organs of their blood supply. Over the years pieces of the heart, brain, kidneys, and other organs die. We get prematurely old and die early in life.

It is important to control cholesterol late in life, but if we are to receive maximum benefit, we must start when we are children. Hardening of the arteries begins in the very young and progresses until it kills us.

Can atherosclerosis be prevented? It's present in almost all of the young men and women in this country, but other groups of people are nearly free of this disease. We are going to learn how to be like these other people. And what is more important, we are going to learn how to protect our children from atherosclerosis.

Chapter II

BEFORE WE BEGIN

As parents, we labor to surround our children with a comfortable home; we shower them with more playthings than we can afford; are concerned with the development of their characters; and some of us begin educational funds before the baby is even conceived.

Parents are busy people. Often, both mother and father work outside of the home. And today's world seems to expect more from our children than from the children of previous generations. With all the pressure on modern youngsters to achieve, we are wary of adding additional burdens. After all, as long as their grades are good and they are popular, why nag about their food habits?

Our children can have a life without heart disease and strokes. To do so, they must acquire a healthy lifestyle early in life. Low blood cholesterol is an integral part of living healthfully.

The first step in cholesterol control is the avoidance of obesity. If a youngster is obese in early adolescence, he will probably become a fat adult. And what is worse, he will have a hard time ever reaching a normal weight. He will be doomed to the see-saw life of the eternal dieter.

There are dangers to this continual weight-loss, weight-gain cycling. After being on a diet, physiological changes seem to occur which cause more weight to be gained than was lost while dieting. There are also indications that "yo-yo" dieters run a greater risk of developing high blood pressure.

But, parents cannot begin the kind of program we advocate as soon as the child is born. Unless you have been advised by your pediatrician, DO NOT BEGIN ANY DIETARY RESTRICTIONS BEFORE YOUR CHILD IS TWO YEARS OLD. Even after the age of two, check with the youngster's doctor before you make changes in his or her diet. Very young children can be harmed by a fat-restricting diet.

For example, in a baby younger than eighteen months, skim milk must not be used to replace whole milk. Skim milk has a higher concentration of salt and protein. This can be too much for young kidneys to handle.

Babies need fat for the development of their nervous systems. If fat is restricted in infancy, babies can have problems.

Rapid growth during infancy requires a lot of energy. By substituting skim milk for whole milk, we rob the baby of much-needed calories.

If your family has a history of heart disease or strokes, make your pediatrician aware of it. Discuss with your doctor the age at which your youngster's cholesterol should be tested.

Some physicians recommend serum lipid screening at the age of five. If this is normal, the blood test should be performed again at age fifteen. However, with a family history of early heart disease or hereditary types of elevated cholesterol, the first blood test should probably be at the age of two.

Although there are genetic conditions that cause cholesterol to be elevated, a poor diet is the most likely reason for a high cholesterol.

The information here is so important that we will repeat it.

1. DO NOT SUBSTITUTE SKIM MILK FOR WHOLE MILK BEFORE THE AGE OF TWO.

2. LET YOUR DOCTOR KNOW THE FAMILY MEDICAL HISTORY.

3. THE FIRST SCREENING OF YOUR CHILD'S CHOLESTEROL IS USUALLY AT THE AGE OF FIVE.

4. MOST ELEVATED CHOLESTEROLS ARE DUE TO IMPROPER DIET.

5. BEFORE YOU BEGIN YOUR CHILD ON A CHOLESTEROL-LOWERING PROGRAM, DISCUSS IT WITH YOUR DOCTOR.

Chapter III

HOW DO YOU START?
(The Oatmeal Connection)

Those eggs sizzling in the skillet smell impossibly good. Isn't this the meaning of breakfast? Especially with some protein like ham, bacon or sausage? Don't you need a hearty breakfast to feel good all day? After all, you haven't eaten all night.

Think about this: The American Heart Association recommends that people consume no more than 300 milligrams of cholesterol a day. One egg has about 270 milligrams.

Then there's the fat used to coat the frying pan, and the fat in whatever breakfast meat you've chosen. By the time breakfast is over, you've consumed far more than 300 milligrams of cholesterol. And you haven't even had a greasy chocolate doughnut!

Fortunately, there are lots of options that will provide your youngsters with a good beginning. And they are foods that don't take a lot of time. If you're like our family, this is one meal where time is an important consideration. We all sleep until the last possible second. After feeding and walking our animals, finding clean clothes, locating books and school assignments, very little time remains for preparing a complicated meal.

Think fruit. Your child can peel a banana. Apples, oranges, peaches or whatever fruit the youngster likes is an excellent beginning. Our refrigerator contains a bowl filled with cut-up fruit. We ladle it out for breakfast.

While your family munches on their fruit, you can whip up oatmeal. We microwave instant oatmeal in a couple of minutes. Pour on skim milk, sprinkle it with cinnamon, and you have something substantial.

Oatmeal Digression

This is the first of several digressions found in this book. Points often arise in the course of our discussion, not directly related to the main topic, that we feel should be discussed as they come up. So, sometimes we digress to a side topic.

Oatmeal is made by processing the whole oat grain into flakes. The flakes undergo further treatment until two portions result: flour and oat bran.

Oat bran has a great deal of soluble fiber — the kind that dissolves in water. These soluble fibers are beneficial to our fat metabolism in that they lower cholesterol.

Plain oatmeal also lowers cholesterol; but oat bran has even greater cholesterol-lowering capability. So you obviously have to eat more oatmeal than oat bran to get the same effect.

Cereal manufacturers are becoming aware of this

information; and in their competition for our dollars, they are saturating the marketplace with products using the word *oat*.

Be careful. Besides the advertised *oats*, some of these foods contain things that can raise cholesterol, such as eggs, palm oil, or coconut oil. Be a label-reader. Grocery shopping will take a little longer, but it's worth it.

If you don't like oatmeal, there are other good cereals. We don't usually recommend brands, but we have found a cereal called *Kashi*, which is a superb alternative to oatmeal. It is a puffed cereal made of several grains, including oats, with no cholesterol, sugar, salt or pre-servatives added. We eat it with skim milk in the morning; and handfuls of the stuff make a fine snack when the urge to crunch occurs. *Kashi* also comes in a cooked version.

For those with no time to cook and who hate all oatmeal and cereals, think of muffins.

Oat bran makes terrific muffins. Muffins are portable. They can be pushed into a hand as a child runs for the school bus.

OAT BRAN MUFFINS AND VARIATIONS
A Basic Recipe

1-1/2 cups oat bran

3/4 cup skim milk

2 egg whites

1 tablespoon baking powder

3 teaspoons cinnamon

1/4 cup honey

Preheat the oven to 400 degrees. Beat the egg whites until they are frothy. Then add the milk to the egg whites. Mix the bran and cinnamon together; add this mixture to the milk and egg whites. Don't beat the mixtures together, just blend them. Now line your muffin pans with paper baking cups. Pour in the batter. The cups should be about two-thirds full. Bake for approximately fifteen minutes. The muffins will be golden brown. If you put a cake tester or toothpick into the center of each muffin, it will come out clean if the muffin is done.

You can do a lot with a basic oat bran muffin recipe. Just add 1/4 to 1/2 cup raisins, dates, or whatever fruit is popular in your home. A mashed up ripe banana is a frequent addition in our home. 1/4 cup of sugar-free applesauce is another pleasant choice.

Chapter IV

LET'S EAT OUT
(without clogging up our arteries)

The average American eats out 2.6 times a week. If you stop this typical person on the street, and ask about his or her favorite diversion with friends, you'll find that recreational dining is at the top of the list.

Critical decisions are made at a restaurant table. There are business dinners, corporate luncheons, and power breakfasts. Even financial journals feature articles on what to order when breaking bread with the boss.

And so a bright new restaurant is a real find. We can hardly wait to tell our friends the news: "Listen, Joe, there's this fantastic place. While you're waiting in line, Koala bears serve wine in peanut butter cups, and as soon as you sit down, you get the house appetizer — curried asparagus tips with pomegranate seeds — free! And when you see their dessert cart..."

Yes indeed, we are surrounded by temptations to eat out. Ads fill our magazines, newspapers, buses and subway cars, and flyers are crammed under our windshield wiper blades. Our radios talk to us about places to eat. Critics rate them, and if our companions haven't ferreted out new establishments, those critics will lead us to them. Each second, twenty-four hours a day, someone is watching a television commercial where the cameras pan provocatively over glorious displays of food. It's a tough world out there.

So before we can teach our children how to eat out defensively, we must learn to do it ourselves.

Don't get discouraged and think all is lost when you succumb to Chicken Kiev, with its butter pouring over your plate. And there will be times when a bagel slathered with real cream cheese is the only thing that can provide satisfaction. Learning to eat healthfully and teaching it to your children is not about deprivation. It means understanding your new lifestyle and realizing that one serving of the most fattening ice cream available does not cause irreparable damage. Your way of life should be one in which you eat well, supplying your body with wholesome foods. On occasion, you may find a bunch of *M & M's* in your hand. This doesn't mean that you have changed your daily healthy food style. Don't scare yourself or your youngsters; keep this important point in mind — *eating a lot of cholesterol in one day does not lead to an immediate heart attack or stroke.*

Now, let's take our children and our balanced eating style out to dinner.

ORIENTAL

We'll start with Oriental food. Typically, this type of food preparation requires very little oil. Buttery, creamy sauces are unheard-of. And instead of hash brown potatoes, you'll find rice and vegetables.

The appetizer section of the menu is where most of the trouble lies. All those crunchy egg rolls and tempting deep fried dumplings! But fortunately, most places serve such things as grilled chicken bits and salads with soy oil dressing. These are good choices to keep you munching along with your dinner companions.

Soup can be wonderful. Somehow we eat it more slowly, savoring it like a good wine. Frequently, children will surprise you, enjoying the spiciness of hot and sour soup. It's as good without the meat, and far less fatty. Get the younger members of your party to taste some fish, vegetable, and tofu soups. If they're not told what it is until after their first spoonful, they often continue until their spoons reach the bottom of their bowls.

Entrees, glorious entrees. The stir-fried foods are cooked very quickly in a lightly oiled wok. Oriental menus are filled with steamed dishes, usually fish, accompanied by an abundance of vegetables. The things to be wary of here are the deep fried items. But if you're craving something crispy and crunchy, indulge yourself at this table, instead of with the fast-food, deep-fried chicken. Usually, fish is rapidly deep fried in a polyunsaturated oil. So, with the rice and vegetables, your fat intake is a lot less than at the corner cardiologist's nightmare.

Japanese food is especially low in fat. Many dishes are created from chicken and fish broiled or cooked in broths of vegetables and protein-rich soybean products like tofu. People attracted to sashimi and sushi are eating very well, cholesterol-wise. The seaweed used in sushi and Oriental cooking is quite wholesome, providing such things as calcium and magnesium. (There have been some reports of parasites. Except for fish from The Great Lakes region, it appears to be a small risk, particularly when compared to the risk of atherosclerosis for those who ingest a steady diet of fatty foods.) The plates are so artfully arranged that they invite you to linger as you eat, appreciating each bite. Eating slowly is important. We know that it takes about twenty minutes for signals to reach your brain and let you know that you're full. So anything that helps you to eat more slowly lets you get full faster and take in less food. Just remember to go easy on the deep-fried tempura entrees.

Even if you or your children wanted to hit the whipped cream for dessert, you couldn't do it here. Just look down that dessert column: fresh fruit, ices, sherbet. Although a few places are picking up our Western eating habits and importing ice creams and pastries, stick to the fruit. Remember, you've just had a bountiful meal, in quality and in quantity.

INDIAN FOOD

A big pitfall here is the kind of fat that may be used. Indian cooking is delicious, but some of the culinary preparation involves a clarified butter called ghee. This is not a fat that is greeted happily by anyone's arteries. Coconut oil is almost completely saturated fat and not a welcome addition to a cholesterol lowering diet, and many Indian dishes use coconut oil. This does not mean that Indian food is to be avoided. This is a marvelous cuisine, making plentiful use of yogurt, legumes, and vegetables. So, in an Indian restaurant, avoid the fried foods. And ask questions! Let the serving people know that you do not eat butter and coconut oil. In most cases, they will work with you to see that you have a dinner compatible with your way of eating. In made-to-order items, they can often substitute a small amount of vegetable oil.

FRENCH FOOD

The French...they are so good with sauces. Except for those special occasions when calories and cholesterol go out the window, be aware of how you order.

Before you cross the threshold of your favorite bistro, think *grilled*, *poached*, *boiled*, or *broiled*. Your second thought should be *no sauce*. If the image of no bearnaise or no hollandaise is more than you can tolerate, concentrate on *sauce on the side*.

Something magical happens when you say the noble words "sauce on the side, please." You use less of it! Be sure to ask for a spoon, because you will be tempted to consume more if you lift that serving piece and pour from its spout. The kitchen, proud of their expertise at creating sauces, often dispenses a generous portion.

In this type of restaurant, there is something else to keep in mind. As you are led to your table, forces are already in progress to bring you warm, crispy bread and little pots of real butter.

If you are able to nibble a few butterless crumbs as you look over the menu, you're in good shape. However, there are people (like one of the authors of this book) who have a computer chip embedded in their brain directing them to slather great quantities of cool, rich butter all over their bread. Wave away the kitchen's envoy before he gets within three feet of your table.

This is another place where you must ask questions and work with your waiter or waitress. Tell them you are avoiding butter and cream. Remember, the chef can do wonders with wine, onions, tomatoes, vegetables of the season, and that glorious little bulb of garlic. Frequently, the kitchen can substitute vegetable oil (in small quantities, of course). French-trained chefs can do great things with poached fish, so make this a consideration as you read the menu.

If something like au gratin potatoes is included with your entree, don't just shrug your shoulders and feel you can't do anything.

Don't be trapped into thinking, It's included with my dinner. Communicate with your waiter. Let him or her know that you would prefer to substitute an extra order of steamed broccoli.

This is a wonderful lesson for the children. They hear the polite communication between you and the restaurant staff. Your example is an opportunity for the youngsters to learn how to order. They understand that you are careful about how your body and theirs are nourished.

It's also a good taking-off point for some relaxed give-and-take about nutrition. No phones interrupting, neighbors calling, or friends announcing baseball games.

Order your salad with fresh slices of lemon or lime. Just squeeze them over your salad and you have an oil-free dressing. Even if this restaurant has the best salad dressing in the whole world, remember *dressing on the side*.

Watch out for the paté nestled among the appetizers. Many an unsuspicious looking paté is loaded with fats. A paté can be studded with butter, lard, beef fat, or fat-rich sausage.

When the waiter gets that dessert cart, simply remember that fresh fruits are always your friend. Sherbets can be combined to look as luxurious as tiers of chocolate cake (well, almost).

MEXICAN FOOD

The youngsters really love this. It's colorful, fun to eat and usually served in restaurants that are pleasing to a child's eye. These places are as colorful and fun-filled as the food. They are great family spots because quick service makes Mexican restaurants a good option for younger children with shorter attention spans.

Again, avoid fried appetizers and fried entrees.

One low-fat appetizer is seviche, raw fish which has been marinated in spices and lime. If it suits your taste buds, it can be a good option.

Be very cautious. Some of the most highly advertised dishes are those high in fat, like beef burritos, laden with cheese and sour cream. Chicken tostados or corn tortillas can be a reasonable choice. Make sure the tostados are heavy on the lettuce and tomato with little or no cheese. Refried beans may sound healthy, but ask your waiter or waitress about the oil. There are restaurants that use lard in making refried beans.

In general, you and the youngsters want to avoid things that are fried or made with beef, cheese, or unacceptable oils. Menus often have better choices, such as steamed tamales, chicken and rice, and fish and chicken in hot sauces or green sauces.

Many Mexican restaurants have gigantic salads with sliced chicken, fresh tomatoes, and guacamole. We have not taken leave of our senses. Guacamole may contain a lot of fats, but most of these are monounsaturated.

For dessert, fried ice cream may sound exotic, but look instead to those old reliable fresh fruits and sherbets.

ITALIAN FOOD

Eating our low-cholesterol way is very easy in Italian restaurants. The primary fat used is olive oil which is almost eighty percent monounsaturated. So olive oil qualifies for a halo on every bottle.

You still have to wave away the bread and butter carrier as you sit down. Instead, ask the waiter for a dish of carrot and celery sticks.

Lentil and minestrone soups make good appetizers; and tomatoes and lettuce sprinkled with a little olive oil and spices, as well as other vegetables prepared the same way. If you order an appetizer of pasta prepared with olive oil and lots of fresh garlic, make sure everyone at the table has a taste so your breath doesn't overwhelm your dining companions.

Frequently, Italian restaurants pride themselves on their house dressings. Ask how it's made. If it's just olive oil with spices and vinegar or wine, get some on the side. If it's loaded with a high cholesterol cheese, opt for our old stand-by of lemon or lime slices, or ask for plain vinegar and olive oil.

Then, there is the world of pasta. Order it like our appetizer suggestion: a touch of olive oil and redolent of fresh garlic. Pasta with tomato sauce or marinara; pasta with clams; pasta with vegetables. Restaurants are getting adventurous with their pasta combinations. Almost anything is good for your serum cholesterol as long as it's not a sauce made of butter, cheese, cream or beef. Pretend butter, cheese and cream don't exist. A good Italian restaurant is a universe of tomato sauce, olive oil, spices, and imagination waiting for your order.

You are not limited to pasta for a main course. There is veal, chicken, and seafood. And it's poached, grilled, baked, or broiled.

Don't even think about dessert. If little Tony didn't finish all his pasta and complains of a hunger pang, guide him to the sherbets and fruit. The desserts on your table can look as appealing as the ones blocking the entrance. Order a whole bowl of fresh fruit and some assorted sherbets. Let yourselves go and just sample away.

FA(S)T FOOD RESTAURANTS

What can we say? There are arteries that constrict

at the very thought of dining out in this environment. You should make it clear to your children that these are not choices in the mainstream of your food lives.

Occasionally, the youngsters will find themselves in these places. If a salad bar is available, children's sneakers should fly in that direction. But keep in mind that salad bars are not totally safe havens. Tuna, by itself, is a healthy choice; but the salad bar might feature high-cholesterol items like macaroni salads, tuna salads, and cole slaws. Pile on the plain vegetables, and avoid the croutons, bacon bits, and chunks of ham. The dressings can be a real hazard. It's time to grab those lemon and lime slices. If children have to have dressing, train them to sprinkle one tablespoon creatively over their plate.

The cheeseburgers and hamburgers are loaded with fat. If your offspring insists on a hamburger with the gang, try to steer him to places where they grill. Teach him or her to say no to the cheese.

If it's pizza that your child wants to share with his peers, remind him not to add extra cheese. The olives, sausage, meatballs, pepperoni, and ham can pile up his fat intake. Let your youngster understand that pizza is healthier with peppers, tomatoes, garlic, mushrooms, and onions.

COPING WITH YOUR FAVORITE RESTAURANT'S FAVORITE SOMETHING

Baked potatoes are a feature of many restaurants. Crisp skin and soothing insides — such a popular food! With your entree, request skim milk for your baked potato. Just mash a couple of tablespoons into the potato. Add chives or chopped onions and forget about butter. Much less fat than butter! (We use olive oil on our baked potatoes, but have noticed some people turn away from this combination.) Low-fat yogurt is even tastier, but it's not always available. Or try a plain baked potato.

There are restaurants whose fresh baked rolls are so flawless, crisp and warm they ache for butter or margarine. Others have desserts worthy of a Nobel Prize.

You may select a restaurant because you have been dreaming of the house specialty. It may be a dish that has enough cholesterol to supply your entire family for a month.

This situation needs tactical planning. Before leaving your house, mentally choose one item you truly crave. Perhaps the restaurant is famous for its herbed butter, but the whipped cream layered tortes send you into a feeding frenzy. You enjoy the herbed butter, but the torte is a masterpiece. Plan on eating what you desire — the torte. At the same time, plan on avoiding bread and butter.

Let the children understand you have made a choice, but don't harangue them with it. This is an object lesson for them, not a boring, repetitive lecture. You might do this with a quiet statement at the table. If others want the bread and butter, you cannot wave it away. Simply state, "No thank you. Although this bread is wonderful, I intend to have my favorite dessert, instead." The children will see that you have made a choice with which you are happy.

HOW TO DINE FREQUENTLY IN RESTAURANTS AND KEEP YOUR CARDIOLOGIST AND PEDIATRICIAN HAPPY

1. Before setting foot out the door plan in your mind what you will eat. STICK TO THIS PLAN.

2. When seated at the table, let a designated member of your party wave away the bread and butter bearer.

3. Have open lines of communication between you and your waitress or waiter. Don't be uncomfortable asking questions about food preparation.

4. Avoid items with butter, whole milk, cream and cheese.

5. Avoid fried foods.

6. NO SALAD DRESSING, or use lime and lemon slices. If the dressing is prepared with olive oil as the only fat and no cheese, this is a decent choice. If you must have dressing, request that it be served ON THE SIDE

7. If the only potatoes are swimming in fat or cheese, request a double order of the vegetable of the day in place of the potatoes.

8. Baked potatoes are better with low fat yogurt, skim milk, or nothing. Why not consider a small amount of olive oil?

9. Non-dairy creamers can be a disaster of palm or coconut oil. Your coffee will be happier with skim milk.

10. The most wonderful dessert tables in the world are filled with fresh fruit and sherbets.

Chapter V

LET'S MAKE A MESS
IN THE KITCHEN
(But Keep Our Arteries Clean)

L et the youngsters help you in the kitchen. But before that, let them join you at the supermarket, watching as you make selections and read labels. Let's bestow upon our children a clear understanding of a healthy lifestyle. A parent can do a lot of explaining to a child, but teaching by example is an even more effective tool.

Your son or daughter may snicker as you lace up your running shoes. However, preventive maintenance, the concept of taking care of your body, will be a positive influence for them. Your continuing example of a wholesome life of activity and good food shows them exactly how to do it for themselves. Just when you feel you've failed and will never get them away from whipped cream, french fries, and the greasiest hamburgers in the world, you might overhear an earth-shaking conversation. Your youngster is actually telling his or her best friend what that nitrate-laden, fat-riddled hot dog can do to a person's heart and arteries. At the same time, your little nutritionist is smugly munching away on an apple.

Get the youngsters into the kitchen. If you're in a hurry after work, children at your elbow may seem like thirteen arms without the benefit of flexible, firm-gripping appendages, but let them help anyway. If they haven't yet offered to help, make sure they see that you enjoy working in the kitchen. With the family at the table, drop comments about a new recipe. Discuss your idea for changing something in another recipe. A beautifully arranged dish is a form of artistic creation. Talk about the colors in food, the thought behind a meal plan, the structure of a menu. Those mashed potatoes would have looked plain on your white china, so you chopped up green and red peppers. Isn't that a beautiful sight!

Almost any of your favorite dishes can be adapted to be a part of your family's low-cholesterol way of eating. We'll give you a few recipes that will show you how to make changes that will "de-fat" your diet.

FIRST THINGS AND NIBBLINGS

Vegetables are always a good beginning. They are low in fat, high in fiber, minerals, and vitamins. Raw or lightly steamed, they take time to eat, allowing an interval for signals to reach your brain that let you know you are no longer starving. With their diverse colors and shapes, vegetables turn a simple platter into a vivid masterpiece. If your children are small, cut the vegetables yourself, but assign your helper the task of washing and arranging them on plates.

Along with home video tape recorders and genetic engineering, modern society has provided us with the *dip*. Beginning as an accompaniment to potato chips, dips have become more sophisticated (and healthier) as they marched into the center of vegetable trays. A dip does not have to be complicated. Often, the simplest are the tastiest. Just remember to use reasonable oils.

Easy Dip

A modest, but popular dip in our house is a mixture of low-fat yogurt and enough curry powder to turn our mixture a light green. You can add a ton of garlic powder and/or onion powder in place of the curry powder. Other additions might be chopped parsley, scallions, dill, pimiento, or low-fat cottage cheese. For more color, try some finely minced red and green peppers, fresh tomatoes, or whatever else sounds good to you.

Mustard Dip

1 cup low-fat yogurt

1-1/2 tablespoons Dijon mustard

1 teaspoon lemon juice or lime juice

Let your child mix all of these ingredients together. Put the mixture in a pretty bowl and sprinkle some freshly chopped parsley on top.

Portions: 20

Per Portion:

Protein	0.10	grams
Fat (total)	0.1	grams
Cholesterol	0.0	grams
Carbohydrate	0.6	grams
Dietary fiber	0.02	grams

Calories per portion: 3

Stuffed-up Cherry Tomatoes

Start with a box of cherry tomatoes, which your assistant can wash. Cut a thin slice from the stem end so the tomatoes sit on their plate without rocking. Now stuff them with almost anything:

Low fat yogurt mixed with chives.

Lentils seasoned with garlic and lime juice.

Lentil Digression

Lentils are one of those fiber-rich foods that have a cholesterol-lowering effect. They are easy to prepare, so we use them a great deal.

Boil the lentils briefly in water. Use one part lentils to three parts water. Then let them simmer away, covered, in a gentle heat for about twenty minutes. (Lentils are low in lectins, which are the toxins in beans and peas that can cause cramping and diarrhea. Boiling destroys these toxins.)

Garlic and Onion Digression

Garlic and onions are frequent additions to our cooking. Our personal tastes just run in the garlic and onion direction. We were delighted to learn that current evidence indicates that garlic appears to lower cholesterol, and onions may increase the "good guy" HDL cholesterol. How nice!

Another Stuffed-up Tomato Recipe

1/4 cup minced red bell pepper

1/4 cup minced green bell pepper

2 tablespoons minced red onions

1 clove of garlic, also minced

2 tablespoons of lime juice

1/2 tablespoon of olive oil

Let your assistant mix all ingredients together in a bowl, and let it sit in the refrigerator for at least one hour. If you prefer, let it marinate overnight.

Then the young chef can stuff those tomatoes.

Portions: 4

Per Portion:

Protein	1.19	grams
Fat (total)	7.2	grams
Saturated Fat	1.0	grams
Monounsataurated Fat	5.2	grams
Polyunsaturated Fat	0.8	grams
Cholesterol	0.0	grams
Carbohydrate	7.1	grams
Dietary Fiber	1.65	grams

Calories per portion: 100

Salmon Spread to put on "Things"

1 can (15-1/2 ounces) of salmon, drained

1/2 cup yogurt

1 tablespoon lime juice

1 tablespoon chopped fresh dill (dill just seems to go well with salmon)

Portions: 40

Per Portion:

Protein	2.28	grams
Fat (total)	0.7	grams
Saturated Fat	0.1	grams
Monounsaturated Fat	0.2	grams
Polyunsaturated Fat	0.3	grams
Cholesterol	0.004	grams

Calories per portion: 17

Crackers (read the label to be sure there are no bad fats among the ingredients) or thinly sliced rye or pumpernickel bread or celery are delicious when crammed full of the salmon spread.

Your helper can mix all the ingredients for the salmon spread and then spread it on the crackers, celery, or whatever you've selected.

Sprinkle with chopped parsley, thinly sliced radishes, carrot curls, or an asparagus tip on top.

Pasta

Pasta is fun to begin with. Like apple pie, pasta is a favorite of people. Angel hair or linguine are delicate pastas that convey the feeling of lightness we expect in a first course.

Start with a small portion on a pretty plate.

A Nice Sauce

1 tablespoon olive oil

2 garlic cloves, minced

1/2 cup finely chopped sun-dried tomatoes

1/2 cup good quality oil-free tomato sauce (there are several on the market; and by now you are a label-reader, so you will have no difficulty in making a selection).

3 tablespoons finely chopped onions

1 pound of linguine

Cook the linguine in a big pot of boiling water until it is just barely soft. Remember, you don't want mushy pasta.

For the sauce, coat your saute pan or wok with the olive oil. Add the garlic and onion, and saute until the onion is transparent. Turn down the heat to medium-low and add the tomatoes and tomato sauce. Keep stirring until everything is warm and smells ready. Add the linguine and toss it all together. Serve on appetizer-sized plates. You can garnish each plate with a couple of whole sun-dried tomatoes and something green like a slice of green pepper or sprigs of parsley.

Portions: 4

Per Portion:

Protein	11.63	grams
Fat (total)	5.1	grams
Saturated Fat	0.6	grams
Monounsaturated Fat	2.8	grams
Polyunsaturated Fat	0.0	grams
Cholesterol	0.0	grams
Carbohydrate	65.3	grams
Dietary Fiber	3.78	grams

Calories per portion: 348

Another pasta sauce

Instead of the sun-dried tomatoes in the previous recipe, slice sweet potatoes and eggplant as thinly as you can. Use about 1/2 cup of each. Saute or stir-fry along with the garlic and onions until the vegetables are as soft as your taste requires. Then add the sauce and pasta.

SOUPS

There is something remarkable about soup. It is as full of wonderful implications as it is of vegetables and other good things. Soup is a sociable food. Although you may be alone when you grab a cookie, you are usually with other people when you eat soup. And when it's cooking, it fills the house with comforting aromas. You can begin a meal with soup or it can be the entire meal.

Let yourself go when you create a soup. Use vegetables, fish, tofu, chicken, turkey, small amounts of beef (without the fat). Soup can be hot or cold, clear or thick.

We'll begin with a few basic soup ideas, and then you

can add your own special touch. There's a whole world of filling, low cholesterol, delicious soups out there!

A FEW GENERAL THOUGHTS ON SOUP-MAKING BEFORE YOU REALLY BEGIN

Don't hurry your soup creation. Let it simmer along slowly to allow all the flavors to blend. The aroma of a simmering soup filters through your household. Your family will begin to gather in the kitchen, asking, "When do we eat?"

Youngsters like the responsible position of "watching the pot." The very young ones should be warned against touching the hot mixture while they stand guard to let you know if it starts to boil over. You can let older children "stir the pot" now and then, but if you have it simmering just right, you can actually leave the thing alone while it gets itself ready.

Don't add salt to the soup. There will be enough flavor from the vegetables, spices, and other things mingling in the pot. If anyone needs their salt, they can add it at the table. If you add pepper at the start of the cooking process, it can give a bitter taste; so let one of the youngsters grind the pepper mill when you're ready to remove the pot from the stove.

Don't feel compelled to cook vegetables in fat before they're added to the soup. Just allow their flavors to open up in the soup.

Cooking times are approximations. You should cook the soup until it suits your taste. You can also vary the quantities of ingredients so the soup is the way you like it. If you hate carrots, but the rest of the recipe sounds good to you, forget the carrots. A soup should not be rigidly made to someone else's exact specifications. Children can provide good input. Our daughter once suggested throwing some left-over sweet potato slices into a lentil soup, and it was delicious. Remember: it's *your* soup.

Lentil-Vegetable Soup

1 cup lentils

3 cups water

2 medium-sized white potatoes, diced

1 carrot, sliced

2 onions, chopped

3 tablespoons parsley, chopped

3 stalks of celery, diced

1 cup lima beans

3 minced cloves of garlic

2 bay leaves

1/2 teaspoon oregano

2 tomatoes with skins steamed off

Place the lentils in the cold water, and bring to a boil, then simmer for about thirty minutes. After the lentils have simmered, add remaining vegetables, except the tomatoes. Simmer for thirty to forty minutes, then add the tomatoes for the last ten to fifteen minutes. Skim off any scum.

Portions: 4

Per Portion:

Protein	16.42	grams
Fat (total)	1.3	grams
Saturated Fat	0.3	grams
Monounsaturated Fat	0.2	grams

Polyunsaturated Fat	0.8	grams
Cholesterol	0.0	grams
Carbohydrate	67.3	grams
Dietary Fiber	12.73	grams

Calories per portion: 338

Filling, Fish Chowdery-Type Soup

2 cups potatoes, cubed

1/2 red pepper, chopped

1 cup onions, chopped

1 cup broccoli, chopped

2 cups canned tomatoes (if you like tomato-based chowder)

1/2 to 1 pound firm-fleshed fish, like cod or halibut, cut into cubes, about 3/4 to 1 inch

1/4 teaspoon oregano

1/4 teaspoon garlic powder (use more if you love garlic. You can also used fresh-squeezed garlic cloves to taste)

Bring 1/2 cup of water to a boil. Add the potatoes, pepper, onions, broccoli, and seasonings. Cook ten to fifteen minutes, until the vegetables are just barely tender. Throw in the cut-up fish. Bring it back up to a boil, and simmer for another fifteen to twenty minutes. Serve sprinkled with a little chopped parsley and paprika on top.

Portions: 4

Per Portion:

Protein	26.28	grams
Fat (total)	2.4	grams

Saturated Fat	0.3	grams
Monounsaturated Fat	0.6	grams
Polyunsaturated Fat	0.8	grams
Cholesterol	0.0	grams
Dietary Fiber	4.2	grams

Calories per portion: 245

The Collection Soup
(A way to use leftovers
collected over the past couple of days)

Gather all edible leftovers (cooked potatoes, carrots, peas, string beans or any vegetables). It's also a good place for any leftover lean cooked beef, chicken, or turkey. (We hope you don't have any three-day-old leftover fish laying around.)

If you have some fresh vegetables that you have no plans for using in a current menu, clean them and cut them up.

Start with one to one and one-half cups of water. Gently throw your raw vegetables (except those that cook quickly) into the pot, along with cut up onions, minced garlic or garlic powder, scallions, and leeks. Add whatever seasoning you like, such as cumin or a dash of cayenne or oregano.

This is a fine pot to add some cabbage to. Bring it to a boil and let it simmer for ten minutes.

At this point, if you have some lettuce, why not add it also? Simmer for another ten minutes.

And now the fun begins. Add raw vegetables that cook rapidly, like corn kernels or peas. Simmer another five minutes and add your luscious left-overs. If you have left-over pasta, let the pot welcome it, along with any rice that may have been sitting in that covered bowl on the third shelf of your refrigerator. Bring the soup back to a boil. Let it simmer about ten minutes. Eat when ready.

Left-Over Thrown-Together Chicken Soup (with an Oriental accent)

1 bunch chopped scallions

1/2 to 1 cup cooked chicken, sliced thinly

1 large (18 1/2 ounce) can of water chestnuts

1/2 pound bean sprouts

1 cup sliced mushrooms

1-1/2 tablespoons low-salt Tamari sauce

Dump everything into a large pot. Add about 1-1/2 to 2 quarts of water and simmer for 30 to 40 minutes. This looks especially pretty served with chopped scallion tops floating on the surface.

Portions: 8

Per Portion:

Protein	9.13	grams
Fat (total)	1.6	grams
Saturated Fat	0.4	grams
Monounsaturated Fat	0.6	grams
Polyunsaturated	0.5	grams
Cholesterol	18.0	grams
Carbohydrate	22.4	grams
Dietary Fiber	5.73	grams

Calories per portion: 139

Cold Spanish Soup (Gazpacho)

4 tomatoes, peeled and coarsely chopped

1 green pepper, chopped

1 medium cucumber, peeled, seeded and chopped

1 medium zucchini, chopped

1 garlic clove, minced very fine

1 medium red onion, chopped

3 limes: squeeze out all the juice or use 4 to 6 tablespoons of lime juice

4 cups tomato juice

1/4 cup chopped fresh parsley

Dump the tomatoes, green pepper, cucumber, zucchini, garlic, onion, and parsley into one big pot. Add the tomato juice, lime juice, and fresh ground pepper to taste. Cover it and chill in the refrigerator for at least 4 hours. When you serve it, you can garnish the top of each bowl with some thin slices of radish or a few sprigs of watercress.

Portions: 4

Per Portion:

Protein	3.92	grams
Fat (total)	0.4	grams
Saturated Fat	0.0	grams
Monunsaturated Fat	0.0	grams
Polyunsaturated Fat	0.3	grams
Cholesterol	0.0	grams
Carbohydrate	23.7	grams
Dietary Fiber	3.81	grams

Calories per portion: 100

SALADS
(As Exciting as Dessert!...Almost)

Salad-making is a great activity to share with the children. All those wonderful colors to arrange on plates! It's fun to work with red peppers, chick-peas in their earth tones, pimientos, red-tipped lettuce, sunny lemons and zucchini, cabbage and chicory. Then, there are all the greens, from pale to emerald, along with graceful sprouts and colorful accents of herbs and spices.

Salads are display pieces. Brown, worn-out lettuce won't do. Past-their-prime vegetables can find a home in soups. Salads are such show-offs that all the ingredients should be fresh. And don't toss them with the dressing until just before you're ready to serve. Lettuce sitting too long in its dressing can taste "old."

When you hear the word salad, what kind of thoughts do you have? If you picture something good for you, you're right. A salad can be a nutritionist's dream, filled with vitamins, minerals, wholesome nutrients, and no fat. But beware! The villain in this dream can enter innocently disguised as your favorite dressing loaded with FAT.

We usually find salads beginning a meal in a small plate or bowl; but salads are versatile and can even serve as the entire meal. Especially in hot weather, crisp vegetable or fruit salads can make a refreshing and filling lunch or dinner. At other times, they are served after the main course.

Salads can consist of almost any food. They can be as simple as fresh lemon squeezed over steamed asparagus, or elaborate gardens of colorful ingredients.

THE SALAD
IN THE BEGINNING OF THE MEAL

The Everything You Can Think Of Vegetable Garden Salad

2 cloves garlic, crushed

2 cups broccoli flowerets

2 cups sliced mushrooms

1/4 cup chopped green scallions

1 cup green pepper sliced into thin strips

1 cup red pepper sliced like the green pepper

1/4 cup red onion, chopped

3 radishes, sliced

1/2 cup diced celery

Any other vegetables you or your youngster want to add.

In a saucepan place the broccoli in about 1-1/2 inches of water. Bring to a boil, cover, and reduce the heat. Let it simmer for about three minutes. At this point, it should be a little tender, but still crisp. Drain the broccoli well and rinse under cold water. Let it dry on paper towels.

Rub a salad bowl with the crushed garlic.

Gather all the vegetables (including the broccoli) and dump them into the bowl.

Then, mix together the following ingredients in a small bowl:

2 tablespoons olive oil

4 tablespoons red wine vinegar

1 garlic clove, crushed

3/4 teaspoons basil

3/4 teaspoon thyme

Just before serving, combine the vinegar-olive oil mixture with the vegetables. Let your helper toss them together; and as a final touch, grab that pepper mill and grind some fresh pepper over this beautiful first course.

Portions: 4

    Per Portion:

Protein	3.88	grams
Fat (total)	7.8	grams
Saturated Fat	1.0	grams
Monounsaturated Fat	5.2	grams
Polyunsaturated Fat	1.0	grams
Cholesterol	0.0	grams
Carbohydrate	14.2	grams
Dietary Fiber	5.96	grams

Calories per portion: 130

THE SALAD
AS THE ENTIRE MEAL

Pasta is so versatile. An entire meal can be prepared using pasta in every course, from appetizer to dessert. Each dish would be delicious and healthful, and the entire menu would not be boring. Just think of all the beautiful colors pasta comes in. This complex carbohydrate is no longer just flour and water, but whole wheat, artichoke, and spinach.

Ancel Keys from the University of Minnesota studied the correlation between diet and heart disease. One of the things he observed was that Southern Italians had far less heart disease than those in Northern Italy. Guess What? The diet in Southern Italy was based on pasta and our old friend, that good oil — olive oil! (Southern Italians also ate more fish, fruit, and vegetables than their Northern counterparts.) Northern Italians indulge in a cuisine based to a greater extent on butter and beef.

In the beginning of this chapter, we used pasta as an appetizer. Now here it is starring in a salad which can be served as a main course.

The Pasta Digression

We have a lot of fun using pasta in cooking. First, it's a no-cholesterol food (unless it's made with eggs, so read your labels). Secondly, it's wonderful food to play with; all those interesting shapes and colors seem to bring out the artist in all of us.

Pasta is not difficult to cook, but you can't walk away and watch the evening news. It demands some attention.

You'll need a big pot and a lot of liquid, usually water. For each pound of pasta, use about a gallon of water. Let it get to a vigorous boil and then gently slide in the pasta. The water should continue to boil until the pasta is done.

You have to be there to stir it every couple of minutes, so you don't wind up with an unrecognizable clump. During this boiling process, don't cover the pot or you'll find a foaming mess creeping down the sides of your pot, onto your stove, and possibly onto the floor.

We can't tell you exactly when your pasta will be done. But we can warn you against overcooking. If you have to err, it's better to have pasta which is slightly undercooked. The Italians refer to this as al dente. (This can be translated as "to the tooth." It means firm enough for the tooth to work a little and crunch down on the pasta.) So how can you tell when it's done? We keep a long-handled, slotted spoon nearby. Every two minutes or so, we lift out a piece and bite into it. When you bite down, it should feel slightly tender. Another test is to look at the cross-section of the piece you have just severed. If it has a whitish color and the color is not consistent, it may need more cooking.

As soon as the cooking is done, pour the pasta into a colander. Then put it into a warmed serving bowl. Often, when the pasta cools, it clumps. You can prevent this by adding a dab of olive oil and tossing the pasta.

The Something for Everyone Pasta-Salad Entree

2 cups dry pasta (shell macaroni, elbows, butterflies, or whatever).

1-1/2 cups chopped fresh tomatoes

1/4 cup finely chopped onion

1/4 cup chopped green pepper

3 zucchini, sliced

1 tablespoon chopped pimiento

1/2 cup chopped carrot

1/2 cup chopped broccoli

1 or more minced cloves of garlic

1/2 cup fresh mushrooms, thinly sliced

1-1/2 teaspoons dry mustard

1/4 teaspoon black pepper

1 teaspoon dried basil

Optional: 3/4 cup flaked tuna, chicken, or turkey.

We prefer to steam the onions, green pepper, zucchini, and broccoli in a bamboo vegetable steamer for 10 to 15 minutes. If we're in a hurry, we microwave the vegetables until they are slightly tender. Or you could use a medium sauce pan with an inch of boiling water. Dump in the broccoli. After four minutes, add the carrots, zucchini, and green pepper. When it's all boiling again, reduce the heat, cover and simmer another two or three minutes. Drain the veggies. Once the vegetables are crisp-tender (by whatever method you've used), add 1/2 tablespoon olive oil to a skillet. Then add the garlic and onions. When the onions are transparent, add all the other vegetables. Season with dry mustard, pepper, and a little basil. If you have tuna, turkey, or chicken, this is a good time to add it to the vegetables.

While all this is happening, cook the pasta. Then drain it and toss it with the vegetables.

Add a fresh green salad, and you'll have a healthy and pretty meal decorating your table.

Portions: 4

    Per Portion (Calculated with Tuna):

Protein	20.87	grams
Fat (total)	1.4	grams
Saturated Fat	0.25	grams
Monounsaturated Fat	0.15	grams
Polyunsaturated Fat	0.55	grams
Cholesterol	.024	grams
Carbohydrate	28.75	grams
Dietary Fiber	3.89	grams

Calories per portion: 258

Fast Main Dish
Pasta Primavera (sort of) Salad

1 pound pasta

1 cup Brussels sprouts

1 cup green beans, cut into small pieces

1 large bunch of broccoli, cut into pieces

1 cup sliced mushrooms

2 medium zucchini, diced

4 shallots

2 garlic cloves, minced or run through a garlic press

2 tablespoons chopped fresh basil

1/4 teaspoon thyme

1/4 teaspoon marjoram

1/4 teaspoon sage

Place the vegetables (except the shallots) in about 1-1/2 inches of water. Bring to a boil, cover, lower heat and simmer for two or three minutes, until the vegetables are at that crisp-tender stage.

Add 1/2 tablespoon olive oil to a skillet or wok. Chop up the shallots, add the remaining ingredients, and lightly saute the shallots. While this is sauteing, cook the pasta; then toss together the pasta, shallots, and vegetables. While you're tossing, add some fresh black pepper.

Portions: 4

Per Portion:

Protein	20.75	grams
Fat (total)	4.4	grams
Saturated Fat	0.55	grams
Monounsaturated Fat	1.55	grams
Polyunsaturated Fat	1.15	grams
Cholesterol	0	grams
Carbohydrate	97.5	grams
Dietary Fiber	9.79	grams

Calories per portion: 498

Chicken-Tofu Salad

2 cups chopped cooked chicken chunks

1 cup tofu which has been drained and cut up into 1/2-inch cubes

1/2 cup chopped watercress

1/4 cup chopped scallions

2 cups chopped tomatoes

1/2 cup chopped green pepper

1/4 cup chopped celery

1/4 cup chopped fresh parsley

1/4 cup chopped onions

1 small package frozen spinach (Cook half as long as the instructions direct; then squeeze it dry and puree with a food processor.)

1-1/2 cups sliced mushrooms

2 garlic cloves crushed

1/2 teaspoon oregano

1/4 to 1/8 teaspoon red pepper, crushed

1/8 cup vegetable oil (not palm or coconut oil)

4 tablespoons red wine vinegar

Your youngster can mix the oregano, red pepper, garlic, tofu, and chicken together in one bowl. This can be refrigerated until about twenty to thirty minutes (or longer, like two to three hours) before you eat. Then mix the vegetables and chicken-tofu mixture together. This looks terrific served on your favorite greens or even better on leaves of red cabbage or red verona chicory.

If you like, mound some alfalfa sprouts on top in the center.

Portions: 4

Per Portion:

Protein	46.69	grams
Fat (total)	16.3	grams
Saturated Fat	3.0	grams
Monounsaturated Fat	3.8	grams
Polyunsaturated Fat	8.4	grams
Cholesterol	0.113	grams
Carbohydrate	12.5	grams
Dietary Fiber	2.87	grams

Calories per portion: 384

Tuna-Bean Salad (or Bean-Tuna Salad)

2 cups small whole mushrooms

2 cups cooked garbanzo beans

1/2 cup chopped red onions

2 green peppers, chopped

2 red peppers, chopped

1/4 cup chopped parsley

1-1/2 cups plain low-fat yogurt (unsugared)

2 tablespoons lemon juice

1 teaspoon powdered cumin

1/8 teaspoon turmeric

2-7-ounce cans tuna

lemon slices

Mushrooms need gentle, short cooking. Steam them for about five minutes. Cool, mix them with the beans, onions, peppers, and tomatoes. Have your youngster clear some space in the refrigerator and put the vegetable mixture there to chill. Shortly before dinner, mix the yogurt, lemon juice, cumin, and turmeric. Let this also cool in the refrigerator. The vegetable mixture and the dressing mixture can chill from twenty minutes to two hours. Wash some leaves of bibb lettuce. If your helper is around, let him or her arrange the leaves on a large platter. Then, he can mix the drained tuna and chilled vegetables with the yogurt mixture, and the parsley. This should be mounded on the platter and decorated with the lemon slices.

Portions: 4

Per Portion:

Protein	44.05	grams
Fat (total)	11.20	grams
Saturated Fat	2.7	grams
Monounsaturated Fat	2.8	grams
Polyunsaturated Fat	4.45	grams
Cholesterol	0.074	grams
Carbohydrate	35.15	grams
Dietary Fiber	7.05	grams

Calories per portion: 417.50

THE SALAD
AS DESSERT

In some parts of the world, a simple green salad is served after the entree but before the dessert. This salad, however, is not meant to be the dessert. Apparently, this custom buys you time after a meal, when dessert is on the way. While your dinner is being digested, mouth and hands are occupied without your stomach being over-burdened.

But we are talking about the salad that stands alone at the end of the meal. It is the dessert itself, not ice cream with a soaring butter-fat content, or cakes, pies, or cookies loaded with butter, but a low-fat, pretty and sweet ending to your meal.

Fruits can be combined with other low-cholesterol desserts like sorbets. They look so attractive on a plate, most youngsters don't miss daily servings of cakes and ice cream. What could be prettier than a circle of fresh blueberries and strawberries surrounding a mound of orange sorbet?

The Exotic Summer Fruit Creation

1 papaya

4 kiwis

1 mango

1 honeydew melon

3 pears, halved, then cut into quarters, with
the cores removed

1 cup strawberries

1 cup blueberries

And, Yes, there is a dressing:

1 cup orange juice (if there's pulp, let it stay)

3/4 cup low-fat yogurt, plain or fruit-flavored

1 tablespoon honey

1/2 teaspoon nutmeg

This is fun for your young helper to assemble. He or she can prepare the dessert plates and place them in the refrigerator. This allows you time for the more complicated chores, like preparing the rest of dinner or scanning the evening news.

Your small chef can alternate slices of melon, papaya, and mango on the plates. Then, he can grace them with a few kiwi slices in the center with strawberries on top. The pears and blueberries can be put on the outer edge of the plate. If you imagine the plate to be the face of a clock, pear wedges could be at the 12 and 6, and small clusters of blueberries at 3 and 9.

Now, an assistant can mix the yogurt, orange juice, nutmeg, and honey, and refrigerate it until dessert is ready. Everyone can spoon their own dressing over their plates, or a dollop can be placed in the center of each dessert.

Portions: 6

Per Portion:

Protein	6.01	grams
Fat (total)	2.1	grams
Saturated Fat	0.5	grams
Monounsaturated Fat	0.4	grams
Polyunsaturated Fat	0.5	grams
Cholesterol	0.002	grams
Carbohydrate	66.3	grams
Dietary Fiber	7.2	grams

Calories per portion: 274

Papaya and Mango Digression

We live in Florida, so the papaya is a common fruit. And, of course, all Floridians know how to prepare it. A papaya starts life with a green skin, which becomes yellow when it ripens. Slice the ends off each papaya. Peel with a knife, and cut the fruit in half. Scoop out the seeds with a spoon, and each half can then be sliced.

As far as mangoes are concerned, this creamy fruit must be handled with care by some people who are allergic to the skin and may develop rashes if their skin contacts mango skin. When a mango is ready to eat, it turns yellow-orange with a reddish tinge. To handle this fruit more easily make two lengthwise slices, carving out a section which is about one-fourth of the fruit. Peel this quarter and then slice down to the pit. This creates lengthwise slices which can be easily pulled away from the pit. Do the same with the other quarters of the fruit.

We-Love-This-Combination-Dessert-Salad

  6 peaches

  6 apricots

  4-6 apples (leave the skins on)

  1 cup strawberries, cleaned and sliced

Slice all the fruit and mix it together in a large bowl. Let it find a place on your refrigerator shelves until dinner time.

Another Dressing

  1 cup low-fat yogurt

  1/2 cup pineapple juice

  1 tablespoon honey

  1-1/2 teaspoons vanilla

  1/2 teaspoon cinnamon

Mix the dressing ingredients together. At dessert time, combine fruit and dressing and serve in longstemmed glasses.

Portions: 6

  Per Portion:

Protein	4.25	grams
Fat (total)	1.3	grams
Saturated Fat	0.5	grams
Monounsaturated Fat	0.4	grams
Polyunsaturated Fat	0.3	grams
Cholesterol	0.002	grams

Carbohydrate	49.7	grams
Dietary Fiber	6.53	grams

Calories per portion: 206

MAIN COURSES
(The Nitty-Gritty, or Why We've Called Everyone to the Table)

No beef is included in this section. If, despite all our nagging, you cannot give it up, eat it seldom, eat it very lean, and not in front of the children, please!

An ideal diet would focus on fruit, vegetables, grains, and fish or legumes for protein. We will use poultry because youngsters enjoy it. It gives them a good alternate to red meat. Then we'll sneakily throw in fish and other good-for-you foods.

There are so many delicious, low-cholesterol things to do for main courses that this section could take over the entire book. We will present a few ideas. Then your family can adapt your old favorites to the new healthy way of nourishing your bodies.

Certain items are always found in our cupboards. Tuna, salmon, sardines, artichokes, mushrooms. Potatoes last a long time, so you can usually find them laying on some bottom shelf.

We often get home quite late. After exercising and relaxing we begin to scrounge for something to eat. After asking each other, "Didn't you shop for groceries?" we rush to our survival meal.

Survival Meals

This is not in the usual recipe form. With survival cooking, you do not concern yourself with fine points, such as exact measurements. For this, our only cooking utensils are a well-worn electric wok and our favorite pot for pasta cooking.

While we get out the wok, pot, and slicing knife, our daughter rummages around the refrigerator for vegetables. She may find sweet potatoes, broccoli, green beans, carrots, and celery. She hands her discoveries to us. We peel the sweet potatoes, clean and slice the other vegetables.

Then, our slightly dented red wok is heated, and a tablespoon of olive oil is dumped in. Being careful not to burn ourselves, one of us wipes most of the oil off with a paper towel. Minced garlic and chopped onions are added to begin browning.

Our daughter selects pasta (shells or thick noodles, depending on home availability). We put a pot with a lot of water on the stove and start it on its way to boiling.

We then add our veggies to the wok, beginning with those that take longest to cook, like sweet potatoes and carrots. We add whatever spices suit our taste. There's pepper, thyme, oregano, garlic, and onion powders. We have been known to make our survival dish loaded with curry powder. Wonderful!

While we stir and add veggies, our daughter sets the table. Then she checks out the canned goods for any additions to our survival supper. She may decide on canned artichokes. If there are no vegetarians at this meal, we may add drained tuna or salmon chunks. When we think the vegetables have five to ten more minutes of cooking time, we add the pasta to the boiling water. At the last minute, we add the canned goods, like tuna and artichokes.

When the pasta is done, we drain it. If the wok has enough room, we add the pasta, stirring everything together for a minute or so. We then unplug our wok, bring it to the table, and serve family style. This is a filling, one-dish meal.

For dessert, cool sweet fruit blends well (especially if you have taken our heavy-handed curry powder suggestion). Slice whatever is on hand and let the youngsters arrange it artfully.

If any survival pasta survives our table, we refrigerate the leftovers (it can keep for several days) and reheat it by microwaving.

The Microwave and its Distinguished Place in Survival Cookery

The microwave has a place of honor in low-fat cooking. It is ideal for reheating foods quickly, without added fat.

Fish can be cooked and then served in the same platter.

There are times when our dinner is very late and we don't want to load up on calories, yet we want something filling. So we head for an old favorite, the baked potato. We start, of course, by rinsing and wiping the skin. We then pierce it with a fork (when we use our microwave).

After the potatoes are done (which will depend on your oven, and the number and size of the potatoes), we put them in an oven which has been preheated to 500 degrees. We keep watching them. As the skins get crisp, we turn the potatoes and may turn the oven down a little. If you don't like crisp skins, you can take your potatoes out of the microwave and avoid the oven.

While the potatoes are cooking, we work as a team to assemble toppings: garlic powder, onion powder, parsley flakes, chopped vegetables, low-fat cottage cheese, wheat germ, sesame seeds, chopped tuna, chicken or turkey, or a little grated low-cholesterol cheese.

You don't need butter. If you do crave something oily with your potatoes, you can use an unsaturated oil, or a little olive oil. We have satisfied friends with low-fat plain, non-sugared yogurt.

Throw together a large green salad and you have a light, quick, and good survival meal.

FISH — IT STARTED WITH THE ESKIMOS

For those who are not vegetarians, fish should be an important part of your diet.

We used to think Eskimos had some secret. While the rest of the world was plagued with heart disease, Eskimos had a low incidence of this destroyer.

What was happening here? Was it the cold? Should we all install air conditioning and keep it at 40?

A group of Danish investigators recognized the link between the eating habits of these Eskimos and their healthy hearts.

What did they find? Eskimo diets were rich in fatty foods, but the source of these fats was fish!

Fish oils actually lower the cholesterol in our blood. The oilier fish, like salmon, mackerel, herring, sardines and lake trout, seem to lower cholesterol the most. Even the fish we used to label "bad for you" are getting a better reputation. Shellfish, lobsters and crabs don't seem to lower cholesterol like other fish, but they don't raise it, either. So if you love shellfish, go ahead and let your family enjoy it. As long as you don't pile on the butter, these fish won't have any harmful effects on your arteries. Also, the fatty fishes can help to lower triglycerides.

In this country, most fish seems to be eaten in restaurants. That's fine, as long as you avoid eating deep fried fish. Order fish that is broiled (with a little lemon). Grilled fish is tasty and a favorite of those who prefer their fish with a firmer texture. Other healthy choices are poached or baked.

Don't undo all the good for your family's heart by ladling on that buttery cream sauce, Hollandaise or Bernaise sauce.

Why don't we prepare more fish for our family? Is it because we think it's difficult to cook? That's really not true. We'll give you a few simple recipes to try. Bookstore shelves are filled with cookbooks that highlight fish.

Maybe it's the odor? This is not true, either. Whether it's cooked or raw, you should not be able to detect a "fishy" odor. The odor is a sign of decomposition that comes with aging and could also be a warning signal that the fish is contaminated with bacteria.

Try to find a reliable fish market to advise you. Remember that the best-tasting fish is the freshest. Frozen fish can never compare to the delicate flavor of fresh fish. When selecting a fish, get down to the basics and use your nose. If your nose says "fishy," don't put that specimen in your shopping basket. Fresh fish is acceptable with a mild, sweetish odor. Look for fish that is firm. If you gently press with a finger the flesh should bounce back.

After you've been to the fish market, the fish must be handled with great care. Don't just dump it on the bottom shelf of your refrigerator and forget about it.

After a few days, someone will open that door and your memory will be jarred. It's almost like buying a piece of jewelry. You've spent a lot of time in the selection of the piece, so you don't go home and toss it carelessly in the bottom of your sock drawer. Fresh fish should be eaten the day you purchase it. But if that's not possible, wrap it loosely in some cellophane wrap and put it in the coldest section of your refrigerator. It won't keep for more than two days.[1]

If cooking is a rare event in your house, you can still increase the fish in your diet. The canned goods section in your grocery is filled with fish! There's salmon and tuna. But don't forget about the less common fish that come in cans and are rich in those healthy omega-3 oils: sardines and herring. Sardines have an extra benefit — they're rich in calcium. Many youngsters are turned off by the fishy look of sardines. If this happens, try skinned sardines. Go for the water-packed cans. Even if the oil is vegetable oil, why add more to your diet? Be careful with that mayonnaise. Remember that tuna and mayonnaise are not a combination enforced by law. Adding mayo can raise the fat content of your tuna salad to more than 50% of the total calories. Try adding your new friend, low fat yogurt. Lemon juice, chopped tomatoes, and scallions are low in fat and flavorful additions to tuna and salmon.

---

[1] There is a trick to freezing fish. Fisherman know that if you put water in a plastic bag and freeze the fish in this "giant ice cube," it will retain its fresh fish flavor longer.

Grilled Swordfish, Easy and Marinated

1 tablespoon tomato paste

4 tablespoons of orange juice

1-1/2 tablespoons low salt soy sauce

1/2 tablespoon olive oil

3 tablespoons chopped green onions

1 clove of minced garlic

1/4 teaspoon thyme

1/4 teaspoon oregano

Black pepper to taste

Have your handy helper mix all the above ingredients. This is about enough for four 1/2-to 3/4-inch thick swordfish steaks. Then lay the steaks in a dish and pour the marinade mixture over the fish. Be sure the dish is shallow enough for the mixture to cover the fish. Put it in the refrigerator and assign someone the task of turning the fish over in about thirty minutes, so that each side of the fish comes in contact with the marinade.

After an hour or so of marinating, you have a choice. You can go outside and grill the fish on a rack which has been wiped with a smidgen of olive oil, or broil it inside. If you use your oven, preheat the broiler. Then place the swordfish on a rack over your broiler pan about five to six inches from the heat.

Whether you and your swordfish are outside or inside, your cooking time will be about five minutes on each side or until the fish is firm when you touch it. Don't burn yourself.

Portions: 4

Per Portion:

Protein	30.69	grams
Fat (total)	4.1	grams
Saturated Fat	0.5	grams
Monounsaturated Fat	2.0	grams
Polyunsaturated Fat	0.9	grams
Cholesterol	0.0	milligrams
Carbohydrate	7.2	grams
Dietary Fiber	1.13	grams

Calories per portion: 191

Fish-and-Veggies-All-Together-in-One-Dish-So-That-All-You-Need-is-a-Salad-If-You-Feel-Like-One

4 fish steaks (You can use salmon, halibut, tuna, cod, or swordfish. They should be about 3/4 inch thick.)

4 tablespoons lemon juice, preferably fresh

Rub two tablespoons of the lemon juice on both sides of the fish and place the fish on a platter, while your prepare the vegetables. This is also a good time to preheat your oven to 400 F.

1 large onion, diced

4 carrots, sliced

1 pound of new potatoes, cut in quarters. Leave the peelings on, but let your children wash them.

4 stalks of celery, sliced

1 medium eggplant, diced

2 medium zucchini, sliced

1/2 cup mushrooms, either stems and piece, or fresh mushroom, halved

1-1/2 tablespoons olive oil

3 tablespoons chopped green onions

3 tablespoons chopped parsley.

Get out a baking dish, about 9 x 13. Let your young assistant wipe the bottom and sides of the dish with the olive oil. Then he or she can place the onions, carrots, potatoes, mushrooms, and celery in the dish. Now, the vegetables should be gently stirred.

If you feel black pepper would be a nice addition, go ahead and add it. The vegetables go into the oven to bake for thirty to forty minutes, or until they are tender. Stir in the eggplant and zucchini, and bake for another ten minutes. Now those beautiful, healthy vegetables come out of the oven, and you can stir in the rest of the lemon juice, chopped onions, and parsley. Put the fish steaks in the center of the dish, arranging the vegetables around the fish and between them. It's OK if some of the vegetables cover the fish. Then it's back to the oven to bake for about another ten minutes. Serve it as soon as you take it out of the oven. Even former fish haters will admit that they have enjoyed a delicious meal.

Portions: 4

Per Portion:

Protein	33.7	grams
Fat (total)	7.8	grams

Saturated Fat	1.0	grams
Monounsaturated Fat	4.6	grams
Polyunsaturated Fat	1.4	grams
Cholesterol	0.0	milligrams
Carbohydrate	41.5	grams
Dietary Fiber	7.81	grams

Calories per portion: 367

Salmon-Vegetable Baked Thing

1 15-1/2 ounce can of Salmon, drained

1 cup cooked brown rice

2 slices of whole wheat bread or multi-grain bread, crumbled up into crumbs (probably by your small kitchen helper with well-washed hands)

3 eggs whites, slightly beaten

1/2 cup skim milk

1/2 cup grated carrots

1/2 cup minced onions

3 tablespoons chopped parsley or parsley flakes.

1/2 teaspoon dill weed

1/2 teaspoon pepper

1/2 teaspoon tarragon

You'll need a large bowl to mix everything together. Grab a 9 x 5 loaf pan or casserole dish. Lightly oil with sesame oil or a good vegetable oil (NOT PALM OR COCONUT). Wipe the oiled surface with a paper towel so you can remove even more of the oil. The salmon-vegetable mixtures goes into the oiled pan.

Then bake it for twenty-five minutes at 400F. This is great the next day, cold as a sandwich filling with some fresh lettuce and tomatoes.

Portions: 4

Per Portion:

Protein	27.17	grams
Fat (total)	7.15	grams
Saturated Fat	1.35	grams
Monounsaturated Fat	2.1	grams
Polyunsaturated Fat	2.9	grams
Cholesterol	0.043	grams
Carbohydrate	23.6	grams
Dietary Fiber	3.29	grams

Calories per portion: 275.5

Simple Broiled Fish

To keep things simple, use a fattier fish. This means that you have to baste it less frequently.

Fish tastes better if your marinate it first. Here's one of our favorite marinades. We will be vague about the quantities, because you'll have to decide the way your family likes it best. Squeeze the juice of two or three lemons or limes (sometimes we use both) and sprinkle some garlic powder or minced fresh garlic, a little oregano and fresh snips of dill. Occasionally, we add two tablespoons of orange juice.

Place the fish in a large shallow dish. Pour the marinade over them and refrigerate the dish. After thirty minutes, turn them so that both sides are marinated. After another thirty minutes, you can think about broiling.

Usually, we put the fish in the marinade as soon as

we get home. Then we walk the dog, feed the cats, hunt for the paper, listen to the message machine, and unload last night's dishes from the dishwasher. By this time, marination is complete!

Before you start to broil, take your broiler rack and pan out of the oven. Then turn the broiler to its highest setting for ten to fifteen minutes. This allows it to preheat. Since you don't want the fish to stick to the rack, you'll have to oil it a little. Rmember that "little" is all you need. We use olive oil. We also use our hands, because we can never find those little brushes we keep buying.

Put the fish steaks on the rack (which is in its pan). Don't throw away the marinade. It comes in handy for basting the fish while it is broiling. The fish should be four inches from the heat. After five minutes, turn the fish and broil for another five minutes.

A famous rule of thumb says fish should be broiled ten minutes for every inch of thickness. This one happens to work, so we use it for a guide.

POULTRY

The amount of fat in poultry can be decreased if you are careful about two things.

First, remember that a lot of fat can be found under the skin. Fortunately, the skin is easy to remove. If your dinner plans include roasting a whole chicken, the skin can be left on to keep the meat from drying out. Don't forget to remove it before serving.

The recipes presented to you will consist of chicken mixed with other things. This makes the meat less important in the recipe. Less meat is less animal fat.

The cooking method is the second thing to consider. After you've removed that fatty layer attached to the skin, don't mess up your arteries by deep-frying your dinner or basting it with butter while it's on the grill.

When we speak of poultry, we mean chicken and turkey. Although goose and duck are considered poultry, we, who are teaching our families the low-fat gospel, ignore goose and duck.

In the recipes, chicken and turkey can be used interchangeably.

Do-Ahead-Almost-Fried Chicken

6 chicken breasts, cut in half and skinned (of course)

5 slices oat, multi-grain, or whole wheat bread.

Lightly toast the bread, then grind it up fine in your food processor — or any other way, such as a rolling pin, with the bread between two sheets of waxed paper.

2 egg whites, beaten with 2 tablespoons of cold water until you find yourself staring at something foamy.

2 tablespoons of garlic powder.

Take a flat baking tray or shallow broiler pan. Use a tiny bit (about 1-1/2 teaspoons) of olive oil or vegetable oil. Smear the oil over the pan, then blot with a paper towel. (This is done so your family ingests as little fat as possible.)

This next step is best done with someone's hands. Sprinkle the garlic onto both sides of the chicken breasts. Then gently smooth it over so the breasts are coated evenly.

Plunge the chicken breasts into the foamy egg

whites. Hold the breasts over the bowl with the egg white, so the excess drips back into the bowl.

Place the bread crumbs in a flat plate, and dredge both sides of the chicken.

Now put the chicken breasts onto your slightly oiled baking sheet and let it stay in the refrigerator for at least one hour or overnight.

When you're ready to cook, preheat the oven to 400F.

Bake the chicken for about twenty minutes, until the topping is a golden brown.

Serve.

You will never miss deep-fried, fat-laden chicken.

Chicken in Foil

There are a lot of variations on this dish. You can use different vegetables, such as onions or broccoli slices. You can vary the spices to your own taste.

This is wonderful served hot, or it's good to keep in the refrigerator for the next day. It's Saturday afternoon and your youngster runs in for a quick lunch before he goes back to play. You have no time to cook. Let him reach into the refrigerator for this, instead of a bag of oily potato chips.

> 4 chicken breasts that have been skinned, boned and then cut in half
>
> 1 cup lemon juice, about
>
> 5 tablespoons onion powder
>
> 1/2 teaspoon cayenne
>
> 8 tablespoons chervil
>
> 8 tablespoons tarragon
>
> 4 teaspoons ginger
>
> 4 teaspoons paprika
>
> 2 red peppers, sliced
>
> 2 green peppers, sliced
>
> 8 tablespoons sesame seeds
>
> 8 tablespoons chopped parsley

Preheat the oven to 375F. Use one large piece of aluminum foil for each chicken breast. Place green and red pepper slices on the foil. The chicken breast goes on top of the pepper slices. Sprinkle each breast with one tablespoon each of onion powder, chervil, tarragon; two tablespoons of lemon juice; and one teaspoon of ginger, paprika. Then mix the sesame seeds and parsley together. Smooth one tablespoon of the mixture onto the top of each breast. Fold the foil around the chicken very tightly, with double folds on each edge. Then bake the chicken for thirty minutes.

Portions: 4

Per Portion:

Protein	35.05	grams
Fat (total)	12.4	grams
Saturated Fat	2.1	grams
Monounsaturated Fat	4.5	grams
Polyunsaturated Fat	5.1	grams
Cholesterol	0.073	grams
Carbohydrate	32.7	grams
Dietary Fiber	4.18	grams

Calories per portion: 347

Chicken And Potatoes Cooked Together and Great the Next Day

4 chicken breasts, cut in half, with the skin removed

3 carrots

2 big onions

3 huge potatoes

2 cups fresh green beans (or two cups frozen beans)

1 cup sliced fresh mushrooms

Preheat the oven to 325 F.

Put about 1/3 cup water in the bottom of a heavy pot that does well in an oven, like cast-iron or Corning casserole dish.

Put the chicken breasts in the bottom of the pot. Slice the onions and put them on top of the chicken. Slice the potatoes and put them on top of the onions. Slice the carrots and add them to the pot. If you have frozen beans, separate them as best as you can. Add the green beans to the pot. Sprinkle in some garlic powder. A little lemon juice is also nice.

Cover the pot and bake for 1-1/2 hours. Now, add the mushrooms. Be very careful when you open the pot because the steam can be fierce. ALWAYS OPEN THE POT AWAY FROM YOU. If you aren't as scrupulous about your mushrooms as we are, dump the mushrooms in with all the other vegetables. (We throw in the mushrooms five minutes before serving, so they're still crunchy.) In about two hours, when everything is tender, serve the whole thing. This is another dish that is terrific the next day. In fact, sometimes we create this the night before and just pop it in the microwave or into the oven before dinner.

Portions: 3

Per Portion:

Protein	43.5	grams
Fat (total)	4.0	grams
Saturated Fat	1.1	grams
Monounsaturated Fat	1.2	grams
Polyunsaturated Fat	1.4	grams
Cholesterol	0.073	grams
Carbohydrate	86.0	grams
Dietary Fiber	16.03	grams

Calories per portion: 548

Rice Digression (or if you prefer, thiamine digression)

Cholesterol consciousness, although of vital importance, is only one facet of sound nutrition. Remember that it does not represent the entire picture.

This book is not intended to serve as a complete course in nutrition. But much of this book is written in the way that we talk to our patients and medical students.

We were about to give you a recipe with that famous combination: chicken and rice. Since not all rice is alike, this is a good time to discuss brown versus white rice.

Let's look at the advantages of white rice over brown rice. For one thing, white rice is prettier. It's also fluffier and cooks a little faster. But that's it for advantages!

White rice is created by stripping away the hull (bran coating) and the germ of the rice. This is referred to as polishing the rice. It sounds nice, like it's adding something. But polishing the rice is actually taking away something very important. This very important nutrient is a vitamin from the B family called thiamine.

The people of the Far East became troubled with thiamine deficiency, called beriberi. They had discovered how to polish rice, making it elegantly white and fluffy. And then they started having trouble with nerve disorders like paralysis of their legs, forgetfulness, incredible fatigue, and loss of appetite.

Thiamine is a water-soluble vitamin. That means you'll find it in the watery parts of foods. It is not stored in the fat cells of the body, and any extra amounts are excreted in your urine.

There aren't many foods that give us much thiamine, especially if you're a vegetarian. It's found in organ meats, nuts, and whole grains. Brown rice, with its intact hull and germ is nicely loaded with thiamine.

Brown rice is a nutritionist's dream food, low in cholesterol, rich in thiamine and fiber. It's filling, and combines well with fish, poultry, and vegetables. Since rice quenches hunger with fewer calories than things like banana cream pie, it can be beneficial in keeping extra pounds off. And if you're an overweight, high-cholesterol person, your first goal is weight loss.

Your Basic Brown Rice and Chicken

4 chicken breasts

1-1/2 cups brown rice

1 cup sliced mushrooms

2 stalks sliced celery

4 sliced carrots

4 tablespoons chopped pimiento

1 tablespoon paprika

1 teaspoon garlic powder

1 large onion, diced

1 cup parsley, chopped up

Remove the skin and fat from the chicken. Broil the breasts until the meat is white. Then cut the chicken into 1/2-inch cubes. Rinse off the rice. Dump the rice into a large pot. Add four to five cups of water. Bring it to a boil, stirring occasionally to keep the rice from sticking. Then put everything together in a casserole or oven-proof container. Cover and bake at 350F for one hour.

Portions: 4

Per Portion:

Protein	20.46	grams
Fat (total)	3.2	grams
Saturated Fat	0.7	grams
Monounsaturated Fat	1.75	grams
Polyunsaturated Fat	1.1	grams
Cholesterol	0.037	grams
Carbohydrate	66.2	grams
Dietary Fiber	7.55	grams

Calories per portion: 375

VEGETARIAN MAIN DISHES
(More than a stalk of celery, a glass of carrot juice, and a limp lettuce leaf)

For Those of You Who Like Something Spicy...Curried Veggies

4 onions, diced up

8 little red potatoes, washed, scrubbed, and diced. (Don't remove the skins. They give the curry a nice, colorful look)

6 carrots, washed, scrubbed, and sliced

1 green pepper, sliced

1 red pepper, sliced

4 cloves of garlic, crushed

2 cups green beans, sliced

1 package frozen corn kernels

2 zucchinis, sliced

1 yellow chili, minced

2 packages of tofu

1 packages frozen green peas

5 tablespoons of curry powder (or more if you like)

3 teaspoons ground cardamon seeds

1/2 teaspoon cayenne

5 bay leaves

Add the vegetables (except the green peas) to one cup of water in a big pot. Bring it to a boil, then immediately reduce the heat. Toss in the curry powder and cayenne. Stir. Add the bay leaves. Let the vegetable-curry mixture simmer while you prepare the tofu. Cut the tofu in cubes. Lightly grease a cookie sheet with olive oil. Put the tofu on it, and broil until one side is lightly browned. Flip over the tofu cubes and broil them on the other side. Add the tofu to the simmering vegetables. When the vegetables are beginning to soften, mix in the ground cardamon seeds and peas. Simmer for another ten minutes. This is delicious alone or great over brown rice or noodles.

Portions: 4

Per Portion:

Protein	23.25	grams
Fat (total)	3.8	grams
Saturated Fat	0.6	grams

Monounsaturated Fat	0.6	grams
Polyunsaturated Fat	2.3	grams
Cholesterol	0.0	grams
Carbohydrate	113.5	grams
Dietary Fiber	22.84	grams

Calories per portion: 563

Notes about Steaming

There is nothing mysterious about steaming things. Buy a stainless steel steam basket. (We like the ones that fold up. They're fun to play with.) Place the basket in a pot and add whatever vegetables you plan to steam. Pour in a small amount of water. The water in the pot should not touch the vegetables in the basket. Cover. Bring the pot to a boil and then turn down the heat, and simmer until the vegetables reach the degree of tenderness you prefer.

Sometimes, we throw the vegetables into the microwave until they're crunch-tender. The amount of time in the microwave depends on your own microwave oven.

That Old Standby, Baked Stuffed Eggplant

2 big eggplants

1 cup almost-cooked brown rice

1 cup chopped onions

1-1/2 cups chopped tomatoes

3 cloves of garlic, minced

1/2 cup sliced mushrooms

1/2 cup cooked millet

2 tablespoons thyme

2 tablespoons oregano

cayenne pepper, to taste

1 teaspoon nutmeg

Your youngster can mix the rice, onions, tomatoes, garlic, mushrooms, millet, thyme, oregano, and nutmeg. If you choose to add cayenne, do it yourself. (It's wise to make this a household rule. Until someone hits their teens, they don't add chilies, cayenne or other hot spices...unless, of course, they have already displayed Julia Child tendencies). Then let a younger family member stuff the eggplants after you have cut them in half and scooped out their centers.

Bake the eggplants for twenty-five to thirty minutes at 350F.

Before serving, you can add some extra calcium by covering the eggplant with a thin layer of low-fat, unsugared yogurt and popping it back into the oven for another five minutes.

Sprinkling sesame seeds over the top is another nice touch. Leftover stuffing is good in the pockets of pita bread the next day.

Portions: 4

Per Portion:

Protein	3.75	grams
Fat (total)	0.9	grams
Saturated Fat	0.4	grams
Monounsaturated Fat	0.1	grams
Polyunsaturated Fat	0.4	grams
Cholesterol	0.0	grams

| Carbohydrate | 29.3 | grams |
| Dietary Fiber | 5.28 | grams |

Calories per portion: 137

FINALLY FASHIONABLE —
RECIPES WITH BEANS!

Beans are one of those foods that help to lower cholesterol. They're low in fat, rich in protein and fiber. (Recent evidence suggests that legumes may even give protection against some kinds of cancers).

Robust Bean casserole

2 pounds black beans

1 cup cooked chickpeas (garbanzo beans)

2 medium yellow onions, chopped

1/2 cup green peppers, chopped

2 cloves garlic, minced

3 bay leaves

3 tablespoons of chopped fresh dill or 3 teaspoons dried dill

3/4 teaspoon black pepper

1/4 teaspoon ground turmeric

We plan this for a Saturday or Sunday meal. We make a lot of it, and the excess keeps well in the refrigerator for several days. If you've made more than your refrigerator can safely accommodate, run some over to the neighbors.

The night before, your assistant can prepare the beans. Let him or her dump all the beans into a big pot and cover them with fresh cold water. Then you can put them into your refrigerator. On cooking day, strain the beans out of the water. Rinse the pot and return the beans along with the onions and green peppers. Add three parts water to one part beans. Bring the whole thing to a boil and continue boiling for five to ten minutes. Turn down the heat, cover your brew, and simmer for one hour.

Then, pour off the water. LIGHTLY oil a large casserole with a dab of olive oil. Add the spices to the beans, and mix into the casserole. Sprinkle chopped parsley on top. Cover your creation and let it bake in a moderate oven (350F) for thirty minutes. Bring it to the table and place it on a trivet. Uncover. Sprinkle the top liberally with chopped scallions. Finish it off with dollops of low-fat yogurt in the center and around the edges. Serve it quickly.

Portions: 4

Per Portion:

Protein	19.75	grams
Fat (total)	2.2	grams
Saturated Fat	0.3	grams
Monounsaturated Fat	0.4	grams
Polyunsaturated Fat	1.1	grams
Cholesterol	0.0	grams
Carbohydrate	60.2	grams
Dietary Fiber	11.37	grams

Calories per portion: 330

Brave, Robust Black Bean Casserole

To the above recipe, add two more cloves of minced garlic and two or three jalapeno pepper that have been seeded and minced up very fine. These are added when the other spices are introduced to the beans.

HAVE YOU HEARD ABOUT THE WONDERFUL WORLD OF SPAGHETTI SQUASH?

Recently, our family discovered something new shining in the vegetable bin. The new star is spaghetti squash. We've begun to experiment with it, and we'd like to share some squash stories with you.

Squash has many positive things going for it. This colorful vegetable with the funny shapes is high in vitamin A and fiber. (Friendly old squash is rich in the form of vitamin A which is known as beta carotene. Current research indicates that this may be a protective factor against several types of cancer.). And it's low where it counts — in calories and cholesterol.

Spaghetti squash has a mild, yet faintly sweet taste. This is a crunchy vegetable that can substitute for spaghetti.

At your favorite vegetable place, look for spaghetti squash, which is bright yellow with an oval shape. Take it home, rinse it, and slice it in half. Put the cut sides down in an oven-proof container with a little water. Cover the squash and let it bake for thirty-five to forty-five minutes in a moderate oven, 375F or 400F. If you prefer to cook it whole, pierce it first so the steam can escape while the squash is baking, and bake it for sixty to ninety minutes. After you take it out of the oven, cut it in half (using oven mitts or something to protect your hands from burning).

At this point, remove the seeds and fibers from each half. Now grab two forks and scrape away at the inside of the cooked squash. You will find that the squash separates into spaghetti-like strands. Now what do you do with the strands? If you're in a hurry, you might open up a jar of a good fat-free, unsalted sauce, heat it up and pour it over your "spaghetti." Another quick fix is sauteing sliced onions and minced garlic in a dab of olive oil. When the onions are transparent, toss in some drained mushrooms to crown your "spaghetti." Whatever you do with pasta can be accomplished with spaghetti squash.

Why Not Try This Nice Tomato-Basil Sauce Over Your Spaghetti Squash?

- 2 tablespoons olive oil
- 3 small onions, chopped
- 2 cloves garlic, minced
- 2 pounds of very ripe fresh tomatoes. Peel, chop, and remove the seeds. (If you don't have tomatoes around or your tomatoes taste very far from vine-ripened, use a large can of Italian-style plum tomatoes, drained.)
- 1/4 cup fresh basil leaves, chopped, or 2 tablespoons dried
- 2 teaspoons fresh oregano or 1/2 teaspoon dried

Heat the olive oil, then add the onions and cook them for about ten minutes or until they reach that pretty state of transparency. Add the garlic and cook it for five more minutes. Throw in the tomatoes and herbs (mushrooms are also good added at this point). Bring the sauce to a boil and let it simmer for another five to ten minutes. If you like pepper, add some. Then slip in the pasta and blend with mixture. Serve immediately. (Purists prefer to ladle the sauce gracefully over the spaghetti.)

*A word of caution about life with tomatoes for tomato sauce.*Taste your fresh tomatoes before you use them in your sauce. If they're overly ripe, they will no longer taste sweet. You're better off using cans of plum tomatoes.

Incidentally, this sauce keeps very well in the refrigerator for about five days. It can be frozen and will last up to two months. We make a lot of it and keep it available. We have ladled it onto rice, tossed it over stuffed green peppers, and even served it over poached or broiled snapper and grouper.

STUFF THAT CABBAGE

We'll present a few cabbage-stuffing recipes. These entrees are filling, rich in fiber and vitamins, and low, low, low in cholesterol. Cabbage rolls hold up well the next day. For this reason, we often cook them the night before and reheat them in the microwave for dinner.

They make a full-bodied, juicy sandwich. We like them between layers of whole-wheat bread or secure in the pocket of pita bread. After the cabbages are cooked and refrigerated, we make three or four slices out of each roll (depending on the size of the roll). Sometimes, we add lettuce and tomato to our sandwich.

Some tips on handling the cabbage:

Trim off the stem. Discard the outer leaves.

Gently remove the large leaves.

If you have difficulty removing the leaves, boil

the entire cabbage in water for ten minutes. Remove it and let it cool until you can handle it. The leaves will be less difficult to separate and supple enough to stuff without further steaming.

Steam the leaves for five minutes. Drain them. The thick central rib sticks out from the leaf. Slice this off, so the leaves will be easy to roll up. And now you're ready to stuff with the stuffing your family has chosen! Grab a handful of the mixture and place it on the stem end of the leaf. Now fold the stem end of the leaf over the stuffing. Then fold the sides over the stuffing. From the stem end, roll up the leaf. You will find yourself with a tidy package. When you place the cabbage rolls in the casserole, be sure that the free ends of the leaves are underneath. Pack them close together, cabbage touching cabbage, to keep them from unrolling. Put some liquid (water, tomato sauce or soup stock) in the casserole before you lay the cabbages down, or rub a tiny amount of vegetable oil or olive oil on the bottom of the pot. This keeps them from burning.

And Now for The Stuffing Recipes
Fairly Plain Rice Stuffing

12 Cabbage leaves

1/2 cup chopped red pepper

1/2 cup chopped yellow onion

3 minced garlic cloves (optional)

1/2 cup chopped spinach leaves

4 cups steamed brown rice

Mix all the ingredients together, and then roll a heaping teaspoon (more or less, depending on the size of the leaves) into each leaf. Very lightly oil a baking dish with vegetable or olive oil. You can put any left-over mixture on the bottom of the dish. The cabbage rolls go on top, packed closely together. Cover and bake for thirty minutes at 350F.

Portions: 4

Per Portion:

Protein	14.90	grams
Fat (total)	3.6	grams
Saturated Fat	0.6	grams
Monounsaturated Fat	1.8	grams
Polyunsaturated Fat	1.2	grams
Cholesterol	0.0	grams
Carbohydrate	148.8	grams
Dietary Fiber	9.94	grams

Calories per portion: 691

Buckwheat Groats and Tomato Sauce Stuffing

12 cabbage leaves

2 medium yellow onions, minced

2 cups buckwheat groats (also known as Kasha)

1/2 cup toasted sesame seeds

1 tablespoons olive oil

Saute the onions in the olive oil until transparent. Then add the groats and seeds. Stir constantly for three or four minutes to prevent sticking and burning.

Add one quart of water, along with some black pepper to taste. Bring your groats mixture to a boil, cover and simmer for twenty-five minutes or until the water has been absorbed. Your groats will now be soft and tasty, ready for stuffing.

Sauce

Tomato-type sauce just goes well with stuffed cabbage. You can use the tomato-basil sauce we suggested for the spaghetti sauce or add some things. At the time you add the tomatoes, add any or all of the following things:

3 carrots, chopped

3 green peppers, chopped and seeded

3 stalks of celery, chopped

3 tablespoon of chives

1-1/2 tablespoons oregano

2 or three handfuls of raisins

Putting it All Together

If you like, add two or three tablespoons of your tomato sauce to the groats mixture. Then stuff and roll the cabbage. Put about 1/4 inch of warm water in the bottom of the pot. Then, start packing the cabbage. Pour tomato sauce over the cabbage until it reaches a point which is about three-quarter of the way up the rows of cabbages. Cover and bake for 1-1/2 to hours at 350F.

Portions: 4

Per Portion:

Protein	8.50	grams
Fat (total)	8.7	grams
Saturated Fat	1.3	grams
Monounsaturated Fat	4.5	grams
Polyunsaturated Fat	2.8	grams
Cholesterol	0.0	grams
Carbohydrate	85.4	grams
Dietary Fiber	10.28	grams

Calories per portion: 429

And Now For Something Crunchy
(Carrot-Rice-Lentil Loaf)

2 cups lentils. (Boil briefly in six cups of water, then simmer, covered, in a gentle heat for 20 minutes.)

1-1/2 cups cooked brown rice or cooked oatmeal

1/2 cup crushed sesame seeds

2 small onions, chopped up or grated

1/2 cup peas

1 cup carrots, grated

1 tablespoon basil

1/2 tablespoon thyme

1/2 tablespoons tarragon

4 tablespoons chopped parsley

You'll need a large bowl to combine all the ingredients. Mix everything together. Pour the mixture into a lightly oiled 9 x 5 inch loaf pan and bake at 375F for forty-five minutes. This is glorious served alone.

Our daughter finds it more glorious served with our tomato-basil sauce (recipe on page 80).

Portions: 4

Per Portion:

Protein	13.90	grams
Fat (total)	5.2	grams
Saturated Fat	0.8	grams
Monounsaturated Fat	1.9	grams
Polyunsaturated Fat	2.4	grams
Cholesterol	0.0	grams
Carbohydrate	48.5	grams
Dietary Fiber	10.25	grams

Calories per portion: 285

VEGETABLES (OTHER THINGS TO EAT WITH YOUR ENTREE)

In some circles, the word vegetables is spoken lightly and without affection. They're found on menus under "side dishes." Vegetables should not be shoved off to the side. They should flourish in spotlight because they are pretty, tasty, and creative foods. Don't think of vegetables as afterthoughts or merely the garnish to a platter. You will be rewarded if you think of them as appetizers, entrees, and counterpoints to non-vegetable entrees.

And, please, don't overcook them.

Canned and frozen are so much easier; but there is nothing like fresh vegetables, lovingly prepared, bursting with vitamins and energy-rich carbohydrates.

Green Beans and Seeds

(Fresh green beans are more tender and sweeter when they're small. They should be less than 1/4 inch in width and 4 inches long. Look for beans that are brightly-colored. When they get a yellowish tinge, they're over the hill. After you've washed your beautiful fresh green beans, remove the ends.)

> 2 cups green beans
>
> 1/2 cup sunflower seed kernels
>
> 1/2 cup toasted sesame seeds
>
> 3 tablespoons scallions, thinly sliced
>
> 1/2 cup bean sprouts
>
> 1 clove garlic, finely chopped
>
> 1/2 teaspoon chervil
>
> 1/2 teaspoon marjoram
>
> 1/4 teaspoon ginger
>
> 2 teaspoons chives, chopped
>
> 2 teaspoons parsley, chopped
>
> 1-1/2 tablespoons sesame oil

In a big skillet or wok, place the onion and garlic in boiling water. The water should just cover the bottom of the pan. Let it cook for three minutes. Add the beans, cover, and simmer until the beans are tender, yet still crisp. Pour off the extra liquid. Add the sesame oil, seeds, scallions, sprouts, and spices. Swirl everything around for a minute or two over medium heat. Make sure it is well mixed. Serve.

Portions: 4

Per Portion:

Protein	11.05	grams
Fat (total)	23.4	grams
Saturated Fat	3.05	grams
Monounsaturated Fat	6.85	grams
Polyunsaturated Fat	13.0	grams
Cholesterol	0.0	grams
Carbohydrate	13.1	grams
Dietary Fiber	3.56	grams

Calories per portion: 293

Colorful Asparagus

Asparagus is one of those vegetables that can lose their color if they're cooked in certain kinds of pots. For this reason, avoid aluminum or iron. Asparagus looks better cooked in glass or stainless steel. This is not of olympic significance, but we like to look at our food before attacking it. A lot of our asparagus recipes use red or yellow foods, because they contrast with the green asparagus; so we prefer our asparagus to have a deeper green coloration.

Rinse the asparagus spears. Then use a sharp knife to trim off the hard ends. (Your knife should always be sharp, because finger-cuts are more likely to happen when knives are dull.) To get rid of the tough parts of the asparagus, make your slice where the color becomes a darker green.

> 30 stalks fresh asparagus. (You can use two 10-ounce packages of frozen asparagus. Cook it a couple of minutes less than the package directions.)
>
> 2 tablespoons pimiento, diced

1/2 green pepper, chopped

1/2 red pepper, chopped

3 tablespoons sweet onion, diced

1/2 teaspoon tarragon, or to taste

1/2 teaspoon marjoram, or to taste

2 teaspoons lemon juice

1/4 to 1/2 teaspoon black pepper

Put the onion and peppers in a skillet (with some black pepper to taste) with 1/2 cup water. Bring to a boil. Add the lemon juice, cover and simmer five to seven minutes. Add the asparagus and simmer for ten more minutes. Before serving, add the pimiento and spices and mix together in the skillet for a minute.

Portions: 4

  Per Portion:

Protein	4.58	grams
Fat (total)	0.5	grams
Saturated Fat	0.2	grams
Monounsaturated Fat	0.0	grams
Polyunsaturated Fat	0.3	grams
Cholesterol	0.0	grams
Carbohydrate	9.1	grams
Dietary Fiber	5.07	grams

Calories per portion: 44

Caulifower, Carrots and Mint

3 carrots, cleaned and cut into 1/4 inch slices

1 medium to large head of cauliflower, broken into florets

1 clove garlic, chopped up very fine

1/2 cup mint leaves, chopped

2 tablespoons lemon juice

Black pepper to taste

Steam the cauliflower and carrots separately, until they are still crisp, but tender. Then toss everything together and serve. This is good refrigerated. It also tastes good made the night before and heated before dinner. The flavors have more time to meld.

Portions: 4

Per Portion:

Protein	2.75	grams
Fat (total)	0.2	grams
Saturated Fat	0.0	grams
Monounsaturated Fat	0.0	grams
Polyunsaturated Fat	0.2	grams
Cholesterol	0.0	grams
Carbohydrate	11.3	grams
Dietary Fiber	5.17	grams

Calories per portion: 53

Easy, Healthy, Spicy Butternut Squash

(When you shop for butternut squash, look for one that is "tan" in color. This is a less colorful squash, but it is one of our favorites.)

2 butternut squashes

The easiest way to prepare the squash is to steam them. You can use a big pot with a wire steaming rack or a collapsible vegetable steamer.

1/4 teaspoon ground cardamon

1/2 teaspoon cinnamon

1/4 teaspoon allspice

1/4 teaspoon ginger

2 teaspoons anise seed, crushed

1/2 teaspoons nutmeg

2 tablespoons orange juice

After the squash have been steamed, cut them in half and scoop out the seeds. Then mash the squash pulp with the spices. This also tastes good without any spice. We like to put the mashed pulp back into the squash halves for serving.

Portions: 4

Per Portion:

Protein	2.14	grams
Fat (total)	1.1	grams
Saturated Fat	0.2	grams
Monounsaturated Fat	0.0	grams
Polyunsaturated Fat	0.2	grams
Cholesterol	0.0	grams
Carbohydrate	10.1	grams

Dietary Fiber   1.45   grams

Calories per portion: 44

Quick, Broiled Eggplant Slices

(When you're broiling a vegetable, slice it very thin. In this way, a lot of surface area is exposed to the heat, so it cooks more quickly and does not dry out. When shopping, look for eggplants that are shiny and deep purple. Once they get that dull, brown-tinged look, they've had their day in the sun and will certainly taste like it.)

    1 very large beautiful eggplant

    1 teaspoon thyme

    1 teaspoon tarragon

    1 bunch fresh coriander, finely chopped, or
        2 tablespoons ground coriander

    3 tablespoons lemon juice

    1-1/2 teaspoons olive oil

Wash the eggplant and slice into pieces 1/2-inch thick. Mix together the other ingredients. Lay the eggplant in a platter and brush half the mixture on the slices. This can be refrigerated while the rest of the meal is prepared. About ten minutes before you plan to broil the eggplant, turn the slices over and brush the remainder of the spice mixture on the other sides. Place the broiler rack about five inches below the heating unit and preheat the broiler. Broil on each side for five minutes. If you want to add a sauce and give the eggplant a pizza-like effect, you can use a plain tomato sauce or our tomato-basil sauce (recipe on page 80). If you decide to add a topping, cook the eggplant two or three minutes on the second side, then add the sauce and broil it for another two minutes or until the sauce begins to "bubble." This is not something you can throw in the oven and walk away from. If you don't add topping, watch for browning of the eggplant slices. When one side looks brown, it's time to turn it over and brown the other side.

Portions: 4

Per Portion:

Protein	0.88	grams
Fat (total)	5.4	grams
Saturated Fat	0.7	grams
Monounsaturated Fat	3.9	grams
Polyunsaturated Fat	0.5	grams
Cholesterol	0.0	grams
Carbohydrate	5.7	grams
Dietary Fiber	1.46	grams

Calories per portion: 72

Spinach and Rice and Things

(When you select fresh spinach, the leaves should be brightly colored. Let the yellowish, spotty, sagging leaves stay in the display case. Fresh spinach is fragile and shouldn't be stored in your refrigerator for more than two days. After that, the flavor begins to disappears)

Spinach stems are tough and can ruin the flavor of any creation. They're not hard to pull off once you have the knack. Fold the spinach leaf in half so that the shiny surfaces touch each other. Then grab the stem and yank it toward the leaf. It strips away from the leaf, leaving you with stemless, tasty leaves. When you rinse the spinach, avoid a colander, because the grit settles back onto the leaves. Use a pot of cold water and dunk the leaves a few times. Change the water and dunk them again.

  1 large bunch fresh spinach

  1 large onion, diced

  1 clove garlic, minced

  1 cup diced celery

  1 5 ounce can water chestnuts, drained

  4 cups cooked brown rice

  1/2 cup toasted sunflower seeds

  2 tablespoons lemon juice

  1/2 teaspoon pepper

  1-1/2 tablespoons sesame oil

  whole wheat bread crumbs

Boil the spinach leaves for one to two minutes, or steam them for six minutes. Saute the onion, garlic, and celery in the sesame oil until the onion is transparent. Mix together the spinach, onion combination, water chestnuts, rice, sunflower seeds, and pepper. Dump it all into an oven proof container that has been very lightly oiled with sesame oil. Sprinkle the bread crumbs on top and bake in a 350F oven for fifteen minutes. This is another one of those dishes that is good made a day ahead. Just reheat at dinner time.

In this way, we can spring spinach on guests who have childhood memories of sandy-tasting, flavorless green stuff.

Portions: 4

Per Portion:

Protein	16.75	grams
Fat (total)	22.1	grams
Saturated Fat	3.2	grams
Monounsaturated Fat	6.0	grams
Polyunsaturated Fat	11.9	grams
Cholesterol	0.001	grams
Carbohydrate	90.8	grams
Dietary Fiber	12.20	grams

Calories per portion: 616

A Sweet Side Dish —
Sweet Potatoes and Apples

Sweet potatoes are not used as much as they deserve to be. We have type-cast them as a holiday food, so they're more likely to be found as part of a Thanksgiving dinner.

When we picture them on the table, we see a gorgeous casserole topped with marshmallows and pecans, and our weight conscious inner voice warns, "Fattening!" This is unfair to sweet potatoes. Those marshmallows, pecans, and butter have given them an undeserved reputation.

Sweet potatoes are rich in carbohydrates, fiber, and beta-carotene (vegetable form of vitamin A); and they are low in fat. Store them outside the refrigerator. If you keep them refrigerated, the inner part of the potato hardens. When you shop, look for potatoes that are firm and don't have sprouts or soft, blackened areas. With sweet potatoes, darker skins indicate a sweeter flavor. All you have to do is wash the skin before cooking.

6 medium sweet potatoes

4 medium apples, cored and cut into 1/2 inch slices

1/4 to 1/2 cup orange juice (preferable fresh)

Soak the apples in half the orange juice. Steam the potatoes until they are tender. Let them cool until you can handle them enough to peel. Cut them into slices 1/2 to 3/4 inch thick. Slosh the potatoes around in the rest of the orange juice. Very, very lightly oil an oven-proof pot or dish and place a layer of potatoes on the bottom, then a layer of apples. Keep alternating layers of potatoes and apples. The final layer should be potatoes. Cover and bake in a 350F oven until the apples are tender. This could take ten to twenty minutes.

Portions: 4

Per Portion:

Protein	3.25	grams
Fat (total)	1.2	grams
Saturated Fat	0.1	grams
Monounsaturated Fat	0.0	grams
Polyunsaturated Fat	0.4	grams
Cholesterol	0.0	grams
Carbohydrate	77.3	grams
Dietary Fiber	8.38	grams

Calories per portion: 311

Sprinkled Broccoli

(When you look for healthy broccoli to serve your family, avoid those with yellowish tips. As with the the pages of a book, a yellow tint is a sign of age. With fresh broccoli, the tips of the florets should be tightly pressed together, not limply spread apart. Cut off the toughest parts of the stalks. If we have time, we also peel the stems down from the florets. By doing this, the stems will cook in about the same time as the florets. When you cook broccoli (as with a lot of other green vegetables), use a small amount of water so you don't lose as much of the nutrients. Slide the cleaned vegetables into rapidly boiling water. Let the water come to a boil again, reducing the heat while the water continues to simmer.

To cover or not to cover? Actually, this is an area of contention between nutritionists and cooks. The professional cooks use a lot of water and keep the pot uncovered. They feel that this method keeps the veggies nice and green and preserves their flavor. They're probably right.

But the nutritionists warn that a lot of water allows nutrients to leach out into the water. So, if you want all your vitamins, use the smallest amount of water possible and cover your pot. Just remember to watch that covered pot. Not only will a covered pot boil, but it will boil over when left unattended.

If you use fresh mushrooms, grab the ones that have smooth skins free from pits and other marks. Once you get them, use them within two days, because they lose their flavor quickly. Wash them right before you use them. Cut off the bottoms of the stems. Don't let them sit around and soak; they become soggy very quickly. However, we often keep cans of mushrooms around, because we like them so much we feel canned mushrooms are better than no mushrooms.)

3 pounds of luscious green broccoli

1 pound of fresh mushrooms (or a couple of
    small cans, well drained), sliced

1 cup peas, either fresh or frozen

1 red pepper, finely chopped

4 tablespoons orange juice

1 teaspoon nutmeg

3/4 teaspoons cardamom

Cook up the broccoli. We don't cook it for longer than ten minutes, because we like it crunchy. Steam the peas and peppers together. Two minutes before they're done, throw in the sliced mushrooms. If you're using canned mushrooms, toss them with the peppers, peas, and orange juice as soon as you stop steaming the peas and mushrooms. Mix in the spices. Arrange the broccoli on a plate and sprinkle the mixture on top. If you like more crunch, sprinkle sesame seeds on top.

DESSERT

For many of us, dessert is often the reason for a meal. And the word dessert itself conjures up visions of creamy, chocolaty, sugary things. This is OK...once in a while. In our society, buttery ice cream, birthday cakes, and pie and whipped cream creations not only exist, but they constantly surround us. Our children are bombarded with ads for cones stuffed with high-cholesterol products.

This is the reality of life in our century. We, as parents, can lessen the amount of these cholesterol cloggers in our own lives and in those of our children.

Don't label foods as "good" or "bad." If youngsters think whipped cream is "bad," there is a tendency to "sneak-eat." When anyone is forced to eat things in a hidden way, they do it more often and in bigger quantities.

Educate your children to the fact that there are choices; and some choices are simply healthier than others. When your child comes home from school hungry, show him a glass of skim milk and a baked apple. Serve him a bowl of cut-up fruit (melons balls, apples, blueberries, and strawberries look gorgeous together). Let him have some multi-grained bread with unsweetened preserves. Fruit and low-fat cottage cheese is another good combination to satisfy that desire for something sweet. Many stores carry frozen popsicles with fruit as the only ingredient. There is a universe of fresh fruit sherbets made without butter, cream, or other high fat items. Fruit juice is a tasty choice. For something filling, keep whole-grain muffins on hand.

But remember that the world will not end and your child's cholesterol will not zoom to 300 if he has an occasional piece of cake and ice cream. Simply let him have it. If you put too much emphasis on the "badness" of this choice, it will become more alluring to the youngster.

Despite all your family discussions and fine examples of healthy eating habits, there will be times when your youngster prefers a chocolate bar. Your offspring will turn down the unbuttered popcorn at the movies. Permitting him to clutch a chocolate bar in his hand does not mean you are a terrible parent.

Just don't let the less healthy foods become staples in your home. Don't let movies and chocolate bars automatically go together, especially when unbuttered popcorn is available.

A meal's end does not have to send out signals of creamy, fatty foods. In our home, desserts center around fruit — beautiful, sweet, colorful fruit.

Just Simply Fruit

There's no recipe for this. Whatever looks vibrant and fresh at the fruitstand goes home as dessert. The season might be rich with strawberries, blueberries, melon, grapes, peaches or apples. And refrigerated shipping containers provide us with intriguing new fruit from markets all over the world.

If we've found melons or pineapples among our dessert fruit, we like to use them for serving dishes. The hollowed-out rinds filled with an array of glistening fruit look luscious sitting on our table.

Introducing your youngsters to a melon baller is an excellent way to get them involved with dessert preparation. Melon ballers are more fun to use than an ice cream scoop.

After you have cut the melon in half and rinsed away the seeds, show your child the technique. Just insert the edge of the scoop into the flesh of the melon. Press down and then rotate the scoop, cutting out a piece shaped almost like a ball.

Then pile everything into your fruit shell or use an attractive serving dish. It's nice to garnish the top with some sprigs of fresh herbs, like mint or lemon or thyme. We roll the banana and apple slices around in a little lemon juice before we mix them with the other fruit. This prevents them from turning brown.

You can make a nice sauce of soft fruits like raspberries by squishing them through a sieve. It's possible to use a food processor with soft fruit, but be careful.

Just a bare second or two will pulverize them; and if you let them stay in the processor too long, you will wind up with a runny liquid which does not look sauce-like. We sometimes add grape juice (unsweetened) to the raspberries, and the sauce tastes even sweeter. If you add too much liquid, your sauce will not be thick. Just a teaspoon or two is usually enough. Our daughter likes a teaspoon of lemon juice added to the raspberries.

Fruits with a more fibrous consistency, like kiwis and pineapple work very well in the food processor. They make colorful, tasty sauces.

Standard Sauce-Type Recipe

2 bananas

2 cups orange juice

2 cups of raspberries, strawberries, cranberries,

sweet seedless grapes, or blueberries.

All you have to do is blend the bananas, juice, and other fruit in your blender until you have a smooth mixture.

Portions: 4

Per Portion:

Protein	2.0	grams
Fat (total)	1.1	grams
Saturated Fat	0.2	grams
Monounsaturated Fat	0.1	grams
Polyunsaturated Fat	0.3	grams
Cholesterol	0.0	grams
Carbohydrate	33.5	grams
Dietary Fiber	5.99	grams

Calories per portion: 146

Uses of the Above Standard Sauce

1. Pour it over fruit or sherbet.

2. Mix the sauce with fruit and serve it in meringue shells (our next recipe).

3. This is also a terrific drink. The youngsters love it served in a wine glass, with some fresh berries floating on top.

4. When you're pouring the fruit into the blender, add some ice cubes; and you will have a fresh, sweet dessert with a consistency like sherbet.

Meringues Are OK
in the Low-Cholesterol Lifestyle

3 egg whites

1 tablespoon sugar

1/8 teaspoon cream of tartar

1/2 teaspoon vanilla extract

Preheat your oven to 275F.

Beat the egg whites and cream of tartar until the mixture is foamy. Then beat in the sugar until you find yourself with firm glossy peaks. Add the vanilla (and a tablespoon of unsweetened cocoa, if you like) and beat the mixture for one more minute.

You now have two choices: you can make about a dozen individual meringue cups or one big meringue shell.

If you're going the individual route, line a cookie sheet with parchment paper. Drop chunks of meringue onto the sheet. Each glop of meringue should be about four inches in diameter. Then your young chef can indent the center of each meringue with the back of a spoon, so each meringue has a center for adding goodies.

If you prefer one large meringue shell, use a nine-inch pie tin. Oil it very lightly and pour the meringue in. With a spoon, push more of the meringue up on the sides so that you have a nice shell just waiting to be filled.

Bake your meringue for an hour to an hour-and-a-half at 300 to 325 degrees. It's done when it is dry and has a creamy tan color. Let it cool completely before you remove it from the cookie sheet or pie pan. Meringues are very fragile when warm. If you want to store the meringues to use on another day, be sure to use air-tight containers.

Portions: 4

    Per Portion:

Protein	2.25	grams
Fat (total)	0.0	grams
Cholesterol	0.0	grams
Carbohydrate	6.2	grams
Dietary Fiber	0.0	grams

Calories per portion: 35

And Now That You Have Your Meringue, What Will You do With It?

1. You can fill the individual meringues with sherbet. The single big meringue shell looks great piled with balls of different colors of sherbet and decorated with fresh fruits, like strawberries, blueberries, grapes, or cherries.

2. Fruits are wonderful in meringue shells. The crunchy shells are great contrasts to the sweetness of the fruit. Little dessert chefs like to arrange rows of banana and peach slices neatly around the shell and fill the center with strawberries or melon balls.

3. See how your family likes sliced baked apples layered in the shell (the apples are baked separately, and the warm apple slices are layered into the cooled shells). Sometimes we add dollops of cool yogurt (low-fat, naturally) or sherbet on top of this apple creation. The difference in temperatures is delicious. (The same concept as in hot fudge sundaes, which will not be mentioned in this book.)

Bake a Banana

4 bananas

3 medium baking apples

4 fresh dates

2 cups orange juice

1 cup cranberry juice

Preheat the oven to 350F.

Mix the juices together. Pour some of your juicy mixture into an oven-proof pan. The liquid should be about 1/4-inch deep. Peel the bananas and slice them in half lengthwise. Slice the apples in half. Remove the seeds from the center and slice each half into wedges. Cut the dates in half and get rid of the pits. Then slice each half lengthwise into strips.

Arrange the bananas in one layer along the bottom of the pan, sitting in the juice. Scatter the apples and date slivers along the top. Bake for twenty minutes. Keep basting. When the bananas and apples are soft, "Bake a Banana" is ready for your dessert course.

Portions: 4

Per Portion:

Protein	2.45	grams
Fat (total)	2.0	grams
Saturated Fat	0.3	grams
Monounsaturated Fat	0.1	grams
Polyunsaturated Fat	0.4	grams
Cholesterol	0.0	grams
Carbohydrate	97.1	grams
Dietary Fiber	6.46	grams

Calories per portion: 398

Dessert Pouches

4 medium baking apples

4 medium or large pears (about the same size as the apples)

4 tablespoons wheat germ

4 tablespoons raisins

1 teaspoon cinnamon

1/2 teaspoon vanilla

1/4 teaspoon ground cloves

1/2 cup orange juice

Cut the apples in half and remove the seeds.

Cut the pears in half and remove the cores.

Mix the wheat germ, raisins, cinnamon, vanilla and cloves. Put some of this mixture into each pear and each apple cavity. Place one filled pear half and one filled apple half next to each other on a piece of aluminum foil that is large enough to fold over the fruits. Drizzle some orange juice over each filled fruit half. Then gather up the edges of the foil, completely wrapping up the fruit, so the centers of the pear and apple cavities are brought together. (Don't worry if some of the stuffing falls out and stays in the foil.)

Bake the fruit pouches for about thirty-five minutes, or until the fruits feel soft.

Be careful when you open them so the steam doesn't smack you in the face.

Portions: 4

Per Portion:

Protein	3.38	grams
Fat (total)	2.3	grams
Saturated Fat	0.2	grams
Monounsaturated Fat	0.1	grams
Polyunsaturated Fat	0.5	grams
Cholesterol	0.0	grams
Carbohydrate	86.1	grams
Dietary Fiber	11.26	grams

Calories per portion: 347

It Tastes Buttery and Creamy, But Isn't

This is so simple that when you tell people how you made it, they always think you left out an ingredient or two.

1 package of gelatin, the fruit-flavored kind

1 cup of low-fat yogurt

Assemble the gelatin according to the directions on the package and let it stay in the refrigerator until it starts to set. Now your young assistant can stir the yogurt into the gelatin and return it to the refrigerator until it is completely set.

We think this works best if you use the same flavors of gelatin and yogurt.

How beautiful this looks in lovely goblets topped with fresh fruit chunks or berries!

Portions: 4

Per Portion:

Protein	6.0	grams
Fat (total)	1.0	grams
Saturated Fat	0.6	grams
Monounsaturated Fat	0.3	grams
Polyunsaturated	0.0	grams
Cholesterol	0.004	grams
Carbohydrate	4.0	grams
Dietary Fiber	0.0	grams

Calories per portion: 49

Chapter VI

WORDS

The first chapters gave you some tips on changing the lifestyle of your child. There was also many pages of useful recipes. Up to now, the information we gave was not supported by any evidence. The following chapters will be a bit more technical. This chapter will deal with definitions of some terms bandied about in our newspapers.

We will discuss lipids, cholesterol, high density lipoproteins, low density lipoproteins, and saturated fats. For the sake of simplicity we will use terms such as heart attack rather than myocardial infarction, but sometimes we must use the medical terms for the sake of accuracy.

In discussing how drugs affect cholesterol it is traditional to use the generic names. Some of these generic names are unfamiliar and cumbersome so in this book we use the generic name only when it is well known; otherwise we use brand names. Occasionally, we cannot use the brand names because the drug may be manufactured by several companies under different brand names.

The very last part of the book has a glossary and a listing of the contents of foods. You may need to refer to those sections from time to time. For those with an insatiable thirst for knowledge, there is a list of references for further reading.

Before we talk about risk and behavior modification, you should become familiar with a few basic terms. You need to learn the meaning of HDL, LDL, and apoprotein to better understand the chapters that deal with risk. Don't let long medical terms scare you. Most are only strings of simpler words stuck together. For instance, *Hypertriglyceridemia* can be broken up as follows: *Hyper-* means high, *triglyceride* is a certain fatty substance in the blood, and *-emia* indicates blood. If you put it all together, *hypertriglyceridemia* means an abnormally large amount of triglycerides in the blood.

The substances we will be talking about are all lipids. Lipid is a term applied to any so called fatty substance present in animals or vegetables. Lipid is really defined by what it dissolves in. Lipids dissolve in solvents like gasoline or benzene rather than water.

Cholesterol is a lipid. It is also essential for life. Your body makes many hormones and other essential substances from cholesterol. So in small amounts, cholesterol is essential for life. In larger amounts it causes hardening of the arteries, or arteriosclerosis.

Cholesterol combines with other natural substances to form clumps called plaques that grow on the inside of blood vessel walls. These plaques take up room where blood would normally flow. They are much like the scale in your water pipes at home. As scale accumulates, it gradually dams up water to a trickle. In time you may get no water at all.

Similarly arteriosclerosis cuts off the blood supply to organs such as brain, heart, and kidneys. As the vessel becomes narrower, there is a gradual decrease in the supply of blood. A blood clot can form in these narrow areas and completely block the blood supply. Without blood these organs die.

If a piece of heart dies, medical people call it a myocardial infarction. The layman calls it a heart attack. If a piece of brain dies, it is called a stroke. All the organs can be affected. If blood supply to the muscles in the legs is limited by arteriosclerosis, walking only a few feet may cause pain.

Arteriosclerosis is directly related to how much cholesterol is in the blood. The level of cholesterol is dependent on two factors: our genetic make-up and what we eat. We can't change our heredity, but we can change our diet.

Do we accomplish anything when we change our cholesterol levels? We sure do. Researchers have shown that when people reduce their cholesterol by 10%, they reduce their chance of getting a heart attack by 20%. If they reduce their blood cholesterol by 20%, they reduce their incidence of heart attacks by 40%, etc.

For every one percent we raise our HDL, our risk drops by three percent. If someone is able to raise their HDL by 10%, they decrease their risk of heart disease by 30%.

Why should this concern your children? Arteriosclerosis is a slowly developing disease. You don't plug up your water pipes overnight. The disease begins in children even though the blood flow does not decrease enough to cause heart attacks until later in life. By influencing your children's dietary and exercise habits you will affect their fate years down the line.

Often you will see the word *atherosclerosis* where you might expect to see *arteriosclerosis*. Atherosclerosis means arteriosclerosis in medium to large arteries where the deposition of lipids are irregularly distributed. Trying to keep these definitions straight is a real mind bender. Most physicians use these words interchangeably. For all practical purposes you can use either word when talking about hardening of the arteries and almost never be wrong.

Cholesterol is in the title of this book, and it is a key word today; but there are other terms you must understand before you can eat intelligently. These terms are *low density lipoproteins, very low density lipoproteins, high density lipoproteins, apoproteins*, and *triglycerides*.

About forty years ago scientists discovered that when blood serum was spun at high speed, it separated into several parts. The high speed machine was called an ultracentrifuge. In the ultracentrifuge the heaviest parts of the serum settle to the bottom. The lightest part of the serum stays on the top. You guessed it! The high density lipoproteins went to the bottom, next were the low density lipoproteins, and finally the very low density lipoproteins.

Why should we care whether some are heavier than others? *Lipoprotein* is a long word, but it is simple when we look at its parts. *Lipo-* refers to the fatty or lipid part. Lipids are commonly carried in the blood attached to proteins, forming large molecules called lipoproteins. Having your lipids carried by some proteins appears to be healthy, and having them carried by other proteins is extremely unhealthy. For example: High density lipoproteins remove cholesterol from blood vessel walls. Low density and very low density lipoproteins tend to deposit cholesterol onto the blood vessel walls and cause plaques. These plaques are what obstruct blood flow. The protein part of the molecule also comes in various forms. The proteins that combine with lipids are all called apoproteins, or apolipoproteins.

Another form that lipids take are triglycerides. When we eat fatty food, the fat is broken down into long single-chain molecules. These chains are passed through our gut wall, but to be carried in our blood, they must be combined with glycerin. There are three fatty chains per molecule of glycerin, so they are called triglycerides. Once they pass through the gut wall most of the triglycerides are carried in fat particles called chylomicrons.

To keep from being too technical, we will stay away from the mechanisms of how these various molecules are formed in the gut and the liver. Rather, we will discuss how they affect our health and how we can control their concentration in our body.

In scientific papers you will commonly see many of these terms abbreviated. For example, the very low-density lipoprotein is written as VLDL, the low density lipoprotein as LDL, and the high density lipoprotein as HDL. Reading unfamiliar material while at the same time keeping all of these abbreviations in mind can become a struggle. Therefore, we will limit the use of abbreviations in order to keep down the flipping of pages.

The chylomicron is a microscopic particle of fat that consists mostly of triglycerides. They transport triglycerides in our blood after they pass through our gut wall. We measure triglycerides, but we do not measure chylomicron blood levels. As we said before, "anything can change in the future."

So far, we have discussed the five different kinds of lipoproteins. They are the chylomicrons, the very low density lipoproteins (VLDL), the low density lipoproteins (LDL), and the high density lipoproteins (HDL). There are also intermediate density lipoproteins. The lipoprotein with the most cholesterol is the LDL. Below is a table of the major classes of lipoproteins and their cholesterol and triglyceride content.

Lipoprotein	% Triglyceride	% Cholesterol
Chylomicrons	85	7
VLDL	60	16
LDL	11	46
HDL	8	20

To make things even more complicated, LDL comes in different sizes. Smaller LDL causes less atherosclerosis than the bigger clumps of LDL.

Now let's take a look at the various functions of lipoproteins. In the table below we have summarized their use by the body, and also their contribution to atherosclerosis.

Lipoprotein	Metabolic Function
Chylomicron	Transport of triglycerides after they pass through the gut wall (from diet) to the liver, to fat cells and muscle.

Lipoprotein	Metabolic Function
VLDL	Transport of triglycerides made by the liver and carries them to fat cells and muscle.
IDL	An intermediate form between VLDL and LDL. **Extremely arteriosclerotic** when it accumulates in the blood.
LDL	Transport of cholesterol from liver cells to other cells and back to the liver. **Arteriosclerotic.**
HDL	Transport of cholesterol from peripheral tissues to the liver. **Anti-arteriosclerotic**. This is the *good* lipoprotein. This is easy to remember because HDL is the Highly Desirable Lipoprotein, and LDL is the Less Desirable Lipoprotein.

The chylomicrons, VLDL, IDL, LDL and HDL particles are giant sphere shaped molecules. The outside surface of each sphere consists of the protein portion of the molecule. This protein covering is called apolipoprotein. With few exceptions, an apolipoprotein found on one particle, would not be found on another particle. Type B apoliprotein is found on LDL, but not HDL. We say that these apolipoproteins are specific for the type of lipoprotein to which they are attached. Below is a table listing the apolipoproteins associated with each type of major lipoprotein:

Lipoprotein	Apolipoprotein
Chylomicron	A1,A4,B,C1,C2
VLDL	B,C1,C3,E
LDL	B
HDL	A1,A2,C1,C2,C3,D,E

So what! It looks like alphabet soup. Is this really important? The particular cover of protein over these giant molecules is what gives them the properties of penetrating into the artery wall and forming a plaque.

Some of these lipid particles tend to penetrate blood vessel walls, stick, and become plaques. There are other particles that remove plaque from the walls. What determines whether a particle is good (removes plaque) or bad (adds plaque)? It is the apolipoprotein that gives the lipid globule the good or bad nature. This protein cover is important indeed.

You will notice that A1 is present in HDL and B is present in LDL. Studies have shown that if we measure the ratio of apolipoprotein A1 to apolipoprotein B, we will get a better correlation with atherosclerosis than if we measure HDL and LDL or total cholesterol.

When there are several ways to accomplish an end we must consider not only how accurate the technique is, but also the cost and availability of the equipment. Also, we have drugs that affect LDL, but none that directly affect apolipoprotein levels. Because of the expense involved and the lack of effective medication, we suspect that it will be a long time before physicians rely on apolipoprotein measurements to counsel their patients.

There is also much to learn in other areas. You might think that by identifying the lipoprotein molecules HDL, IDL, LDL, and VLDL that we have covered them all. We are now beginning to learn about subclasses of LDL. There are some low density lipoproteins that are slightly higher or lower in density, but they are not so different that they fall out of the LDL class in general. They are all very closely related in density, but may have different properties regarding their effect on acceleration of atherosclerosis.

We have covered a lot of information in the last few pages, and if you want to reduce it to the most important facts, here they are:

1. LDL (Less Desirable Lipoprotein), or low density lipoprotein, is the bad lipid to have in the blood. It contains much cholesterol, which it tends to deposit on the arterial wall, obstructing the flow of blood. The less LDL in the blood, the better.

2. HDL (Highly Desirable Lipoprotein), or high density lipoprotein, is a good lipid to have in the blood. It contains less cholesterol than LDL, but most important, it will transport cholesterol away from the blood vessel walls. Having a lot of HDL in the blood is good.

If you remember only the two principles listed above, you can understand the coming chapters. You will understand why and how you must alter the life style of your children to protect them from the ravages of arteriosclerosis.

We will discuss the effects of cholesterol on longevity later, but first we must find out what a normal blood cholesterol level is. If we take the blood of thousands of

Americans and measure the cholesterol in that blood, we will get the results listed in the table below.

AVERAGE CHOLESTEROL IN THE UNITED STATES

Age	Male (by percentile)			Female (by percentile)		
	75th	90th	95th	75th	90th	95th
0-19	170	185	200	175	190	200
20-24	185	205	220	190	215	230
25-29	200	225	245	195	220	235
30-34	215	240	255	195	220	235
35-39	225	250	270	205	230	245
40-44	230	250	270	215	235	255
45-49	235	260	275	225	250	270
50-54	235	260	275	240	265	285
55-69	235	260	275	250	275	295

This table takes some explanation. Notice that it is titled *AVERAGE* rather than *NORMAL*. Usually, when we measure a blood value, such as sugar or potassium, in a large group of people, the average value is considered normal. Those of us who have had a little statistics understand that two standard deviations above and below the average are still considered in the normal range.

A few years ago laboratories and doctors made that mistake about cholesterol. They considered a cholesterol of 300 to be in the normal range. A cholesterol of 300 may be in the *average range*, but it certainly is not normal.

If we did the same blood sampling in Japan, we would find a much lower average for cholesterol. And as you might suspect, their incidence of heart attacks are 1/50th that of Americans.

In the far left column are listed the age ranges, and along the top are listed the percentiles in men and women. The term *percentile* may be confusing. Let us take an example by looking at the very bottom row. From age 55 through 69, if you were a male and had a cholesterol of 235, you can see that you were in the 75th percentile. This means that 25% of men at that range would have cholesterols equal to or higher than you. If your cholesterol was 275, that would put you in the 95th percentile, and only 5% of men in your age group would have a higher cholesterol. When we classify the level of cholesterol as being 200, we mean that there is 200 milligrams percent (mg%) in the blood.

That means that every 100 milliliters of blood contains 200 mg of cholesterol. Most of the time we will leave out the *mg%* when we give a cholesterol level.

Is this information about cholesterol levels important? Sure! We have already noted that the Japanese have 1/50th the incidence of heart disease of Americans, but they are different in other ways too.

As previously stated, heredity is a very important factor in determining whether or not you will have heart disease. Japanese people look different from Americans and are born with different genes. Perhaps the gene that colors their skin also protects them from arteriosclerosis? We know, however, that when the Japanese come to the United States, they share our eating habits. They also begin to share our health problems. Japanese-Americans now have almost the same amount of heart disease as the rest of us. They still keep some of their traditional eating habits, so their incidence of heart disease is not as bad as other Americans. The National Institute of Health considers those who have cholesterol levels above the 90th percentile to be at high risk. Those who are between the 75th and 90th percentiles are at moderate risk.

However, total cholesterol level is not the whole story. If it was, why would we bother you with a bunch of initials like HDL, LDL, VLDL, etc.?

Many studies have shown that high levels of HDL reduce the chance of getting arteriosclerosis. Total HDL levels average about 50 milligrams per 100 cc of blood. An individual who has a HDL of 25 has about two to three times the risk of the average person. Someone with a HDL of 75 has about half the risk.

Another way of evaluating risk is to look at the ratio of cholesterol to HDL. That is, divide the milligrams of cholesterol by the milligrams of HDL, and use that number. The higher the number, the higher the risk.

Some doctors rely on the ratio of LDL to HDL. Which is best? We can't be certain as to which method is the more reliable. It seems that you should use a method that measures not only for the total cholesterol, but also considers the amount of HDL in the blood.

A major portion of this book will be devoted to how you can reduce your blood cholesterol levels. What about raising the level of HDL? This is not going to take much room, because there is only one practical way of raising your HDL. Except for some medications, only exercise will raise your HDL. You must do aerobic exercise which raises your heart rate for no less than thirty minutes, at least four times a week. By running only six miles a week, you will increase your HDL by ten percent within six months.

Not only are you going to have to control your child's dietary habits, but you are going to have to break him or her of the couch potato lifestyle. We emphasize diet and exercise because these are areas of your life over which you can take charge. Setting an example for your children will create a healthy lifestyle for them to follow.

What other factors raise cholesterol? There are several diseases that raise cholesterol, increasing your chance of getting strokes and heart attacks. Some of these diseases are cirrhosis of the liver, hypothyroidism, and nephrosis. Often with control of the disease, there is control of the cholesterol.

We have already mentioned heredity. This is a factor we cannot change. Certain medications cause a rise in cholesterol. Here the physician must make a judgment. Is there another drug, just as safe and effective, that he can substitute? Is the disease important enough so a rise in cholesterol must be accepted? Some of the drugs that raise cholesterol are: alcohol; hormones like estrogen, progesterone, and cortisone; certain diuretics; and some beta blockers such as Inderal.

You and your children may have been blessed with wonderful genes. Perhaps you eat beef every day and you all have cholesterol levels under 150. Many specialists in this area believe that everyone should be tested for their blood cholesterol level. If you are concerned enough to read this book, you should be concerned enough to have your doctor test you and your children. If you and your family use whole milk, eat lamb and beef daily, and still have cholesterols under 200, with a decent HDL, you don't need this book.

Chapter VII

RISK

In this chapter we will talk about what it means to have high cholesterol, high triglycerides, or high HDL. Many tables and graphs are included, but they will be carefully explained.

The public is deluged with books on health, many containing valuable information. Others are loaded with quackery. You can find books on grapefruit diets, high fat diets, and watermelon diets. How do you know that this cholesterol diet stuff is not just a bunch of hokum? We know the following facts:

1. Feeding some animals diets high in cholesterol leads to atherosclerotic plaques.

2. Atherosclerotic plaques contain cholesterol as a major component.

3. We see obstructing atherosclerotic plaques only in people who have a cholesterol greater than 150.

4. We can associate the blood cholesterol level with the chance that a person will get atherosclerotic disease.

5. The amount of atherosclerotic plaques is related to serum cholesterol and low density lipoprotein.

6. Lowering blood cholesterol and LDL leads to a reduced chance of acquiring atherosclerotic disease.

7. Atherosclerotic plaques have been observed to regress when cholesterol in the blood has been lowered.

The table below is just a portion of the one pictured in chapter VII. We have included only the 75th percentile at each age group. If your cholesterol is above the 75th percentile, there is reason for concern.

CHOLESTEROL BLOOD LEVEL
75th percentile

Age:	0-19	20-24	25-29
Women	170	185	200
Men	175	190	195

Age:	30-34	35-39	30-44
Women	215	225	230
Men	195	205	215

Age:	45-49	50-54	55-69
Women	235	235	235
Men	225	240	250

In general, your goal should be reduction of total cholesterol to less than 200. As you can see, however, cholesterol rises as we get older.

Logically, we should be most concerned with maintaining a low cholesterol level at a young age. The younger you are, the more time cholesterol has in which to damage your arteries.

What level of cholesterol is totally OK? In the MRFIT study a large population was examined to discover the relationship between the blood level of cholesterol and the incidence of death from heart disease. The curve from the study shows that mortality does not begin to level off until cholesterol is reduced to about 150. There seems to be no lower limit to what is a good cholesterol.

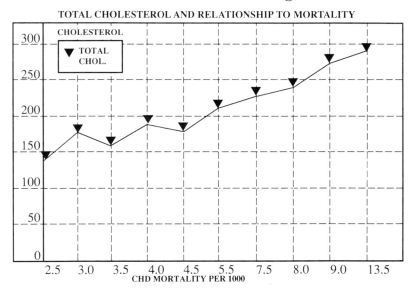

TOTAL CHOLESTEROL AND RELATIONSHIP TO MORTALITY

However, there must be a point where we place less emphasis on a lower cholesterol. Someone with a cholesterol of 170 has better things to do than strive to reduce his cholesterol to 150.

What about the person who has a cholesterol of 265? He has twice the chance of having a myocardial infarction as a person with a cholesterol of 200. Those who have cholesterols of 300 have a 400% greater chance of having a myocardial infarction than someone with a cholesterol of 200.

Cholesterol blood levels are not the only risk factor to consider when looking at lipids. There is a small town in Massachusetts called Framingham. The people like their town and very few move away. There aren't many newcomers either. This is a wonderful population to study. Framingham has become famous because of many long duration studies regarding their exercise habits, eating habits, blood pressure, and other factors. These factors have been related to the incidence of heart disease and stroke in this population. The Framingham studies have gone on for decades. Below is a summary of what we know about the people in Framingham, and their risk for heart disease. In the Framingham Heart Study, half of the men and women who had myocardial infarctions had cholesterol levels between 200 and 250. Those having HDL levels below 40 have the same risk of heart disease as those with cholesterol levels above 300. In a large study in West Germany, 65% of those with myocardial infarctions had a HDL below 35%. So your HDL level may be even more important than your cholesterol level.

How can we use both HDL and total cholesterol to give us a better understanding of our chance of heart attacks or strokes? Since high cholesterol raises the risk, and high HDL lowers the risk, a ratio of the two should tell us something. Here comes another table:

CHOLESTEROL/HDL RATIO
Coronary Heart Disease

(CHD) Risk Groups	Male	Female
Lowest risk	less than 3.5	less than 3.5
Below average risk	3.5 to 4.4	3.5 to 4.4
Average risk	4.5 to 6.4	4.5 to 5.5
High risk	6.5 to 13.5	5.6 to 10.9
Highest risk	13.5 or greater	11 or greater

Suppose you have a blood cholesterol of 200 and an HDL of 25. If you divide 200 by 25 you get the cholesterol/HDL ratio which equals 8. You can see that even with a satisfactory cholesterol, a low HDL can throw you into a high risk group. What if your ratio puts you in the average risk group? Don't settle for that. Remember that up to now the average person in the United States has been dying of atherosclerosis. You must strive for a below average risk.

The answer to the next question seems obvious. Suppose I have a high cholesterol which places me in a high risk group, and I lower my cholesterol. Do I change my risk of atherosclerosis? "Well, of course it's obvious," you would say. If you are in a high risk group and change your level to that of a low risk group, you should share the benefits of the low risk group.

Logic does not always hold in medicine. People are complicated! There are always unseen factors that make simple logic alone untrustworthy. These suppositions must always be tested to be believed. Fortunately,this was tested. A large group of people had their cholesterol lowered. Each 1 percent reduction in cholesterol was accompanied by a 2 percent reduction in coronary heart disease. This means that if you can reduce your cholesterol by 15% then you can reduce your chance of having a heart attack by 30%.

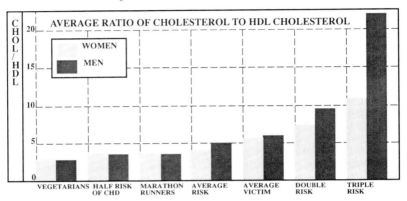

Now let's take a look at triglycerides? This is another lipid found in the blood, and we have not discussed its relationship to atherosclerosis. The highest concentration of triglyceride is in the chylomicrons. However, the VLDL fraction of blood also contains great concentrations of triglyceride.

Triglycerides have a much weaker relationship than cholesterol to heart disease. When we study large populations, the more pronounced effect of the cholesterol levels mask the weaker effect of the triglyceride levels. Also, any medication that lowers triglycerides, lowers cholesterol. Analyzing the numbers becomes difficult when you have so many variables.

In the past, triglycerides have been considered to be relatively unimportant. The normal blood triglyceride level is less than 175mg%, but most physicians did not become concerned unless the triglyceride level was greater than 500mg%. In one study the triglyceride data collected on 7,500 men and women was reanalyzed. Blood levels of triglycerides below 180mg% were found not to be a factor in increasing heart disease, but increased significantly with triglycerides above that level. The relationship is not a simple one. The risk of heart disease increased when the triglyceride level rose from 180mg% to 300mg%, but beyond that point the risk began to drop. At this time we don't understand the complex mechanisms involved.

We have talked about the different settling rates of lipids in the ultracentrifuge. We have divided the lipoproteins into HDL, IDL, LDL, and VLDL. Yet there is always someone who can cut the pie into smaller slices. Not only do we have LDL, but we have small, dense particles of LDL, and bigger less dense particles of LDL. People who had suffered myocardial infarctions are more likely to have the small LDL particles. At the present time, your physician can not test for this abnormality.

We also know that HDL can be divided into several subfractions. Each of which is not equally effective in preventing atherosclerosis, or equally effected by various drugs.

Why do some people who are the proper weight and eat the proper things still have high cholesterol? There are many diseases that cause lipid abnormalities. Some we understand, but others we just attribute to heredity. Below is a list which attempts to organize this poorly understood subject. There is no need for the average physician to memorize this list. Whether someone has familial hypercholesterolemia or familial combined hyperlipidemia is only of interest to researchers in the field. All he needs to know about his patient is:

1. Does the patient have high cholesterol?

2. Does the patient have high triglycerides?

3. How high is the HDL, and LDL?

4. What is the Cholesterol/HDL ratio?

LIPID DISORDERS (N = normal or slightly elevated)

Disorder	Elevated Lipoprotein	Cholesterol	Triglyceride
Cholesterol Elevated			
Familial hyper- cholesterolemia	LDL	300	N
Familial combined hyperlipidemia	LDL	275	200-300
Polygenic hyper- cholesterolemia	LDL	275	200-300
Triglycerides Elevated			
Familial hyper- triglyceridemia	VLDL	N	250-500
Familial type V hyper- lipoproteinemia	VLDL and chylomicrons	N	500
Familial combined hyperlipidemia	VLDL or VDL+ chylomicrons	N	250-500
Lipoprotein lipase deficiency	chylomicrons	N	500

Disorder	Elevated Lipoprotein	Cholesterol	Triglyceride
Apo-C-II deficiency	chylomicrons	N	500
Type III hyperlipoproteinemia	VLDL	275-500	275-500

As you can see from their names, most of these abnormalities are defined by which lipid is abnormal in amount Also they can be characterized by whether it is cholesterol, triglycerides, or both that are elevated. Only in a few cases, such as Apo-C-II deficiency, have we defined the actual metabolic defect. The other fact that is obvious from this table is that the severity of the lipid abnormality can have a wide range. Someone with type III hyperlipoproteinemia may have a cholesterol of 275 and a triglyceride of 275. This can probably be managed with diet alone. What about the individual with a cholesterol of 500 and a triglyceride of 500? It is doubtful that diet alone would do the trick, and this person would need diet plus drugs.

From this table we can see that lipid abnormalities originate from different causes. There must be several diseases that cause abnormalities in cholesterol and triglycerides. We have only limited knowledge about these diseases, but we can see that they cause different problems for the victim. We are also learning about new diseases involving abnormal lipids. In about 15% of people with hypertension there has been found triglyceride and LDL levels greater than the 95th percentile. Those same people have HDL levels that are very low. The researchers who found this relationship feel they have discovered a new disease. They have labeled this disease Familial Dyslipidemic Hypertension. We are sure that by the time this book is published there will be other such syndromes or diseases. We will not have time to include them in this edition.

In the next table we have listed the same disorders as we have in the table above, but this time we show where the harm is done.

DISEASES ASSOCIATED WITH LIPID ABNORMALITIES

Disorder	Coronary Artery Disease	Peripheral Vascular Disease	Obesity	Diabetes	Pancreatitis
Familial hyper-cholesterolemia	+				
Familial combined hyperlipidemia	+		+	+	
Polygenic hyper-cholesterolemia	+				
Familial hyper-triglyceridemia	+		+	+	
Familial combined hyperlipidemia	+		+	+	
Familial type V hyperlipoproteinemia	?		+	+	+
Lipoprotein lipase deficiency					+

Disorder	Coronary Artery Disease	Peripheral Vascular Disease	Obesity	Diabetes	Pancreatitis
Apo-C-II deficiency					+
Type III hyper-lipoproteinemia	+	+	+	+	

Those disorders with a plus sign in the column for coronary artery disease cause atherosclerosis in the arteries that feed the heart. People with these disorders are at risk for angina and myocardial infarctions. Type III hyperlipoproteinemia is the only disorder with a plus sign in the PERIPHERAL disease column. People with this disorder commonly have atherosclerosis involving the arteries in the legs. After they walk a few feet, their leg muscles run out of oxygen because of an inadequate blood supply. They must then rest and allow the muscles to recover before they can walk further.

As you can see, there are quite a few differences among the lipid disorders. Lipoprotein lipase deficiency and Apo-C-II deficiency do not seem to harm the blood vessels. However, they are both associated with a disease of the pancreas. Lipoprotein lipase deficiency causes cholesterol deposits to appear on the skin even though it spares the arteries.

How can a doctor tell what kind of lipid disorder you have? He can make an intelligent guess from your blood chemistries. If you have a cholesterol of 350, a triglyceride level of 250, and diabetes, he can be fairly certain that you have familial combined hyperlipidemia. But his diagnosis is nothing more than an academic exercise. He only needs to determine that you have an elevated cholesterol, triglyceride level, and blood sugar to advise you on what to do to reduce those levels.

Lipid abnormalities occur in several diseases in which the primary effort is directed to controlling the disease. Correction of the lipid abnormality generally follows.

LIPID ABNORMALITIES ASSOCIATED WITH SOME MEDICAL PROBLEMS

Disorder	Elevated Lipoprotein	Cholesterol	Triglyceride
Diabetes	VLDL	200-300	300-10,000
Hypothyroidism	LDL	300-400	100-400
Nephrotice Syndrome	VLDL, LDL	300-500	100-500
Uremia	VLDL	200-300	300-800
Cirrhosis	Apolipoprotein X	300-2000	100
Alcoholism	VLDL	200-300	300-10,000
Birth Control Pills	VLDL	200-300	300-10,000

The last two items listed, alcoholism and birth control pills, are commonly associated with pancreatitis and fatty deposits on the skin. Neither is associated with premature atherosclerosis.

In this chapter we have shown how an elevation in cholesterol puts you and your family at risk of atherosclerosis. In addition to the cholesterol level we have shown how important it is to have a high HDL level. It may be best to combine cholesterol and HDL in a ratio to give us the best estimate of risk.

We have given you more information about lipid disease than you will ever need. We can't expect you to commit all of this data to memory. Use this as a reference, and come back to this chapter whenever you have a question.

All you really have to know is that high blood cholesterol and triglyceride is bad and that high blood HDL is good.

You shouldn't get the idea that lipids are the only risk factors in vascular disease. Several others are also very important. They are smoking (which is devastating), heredity, being a male, age itself, and a sedentary life. We haven't talked much about these other factors because this book is about cholesterol. We will discuss exercise later, because it has some important effects in regard to cholesterol.

If you are a male, there is not much you can do about it. If you were born from parents, one or both of who died in their 40s of heart disease, adoption is no solution. So you are left with only smoking, exercise, and diet as factors under your control.

Chapter VIII

CONTROL

In this chapter we will teach you techniques of healthy living. A healthy lifestyle will help assure you of relative freedom from strokes and heart attacks. But some limitations must be kept in mind.

The low fat diet is not healthy for infants. An infant's nutritional requirements include fats for normal weight gain and brain development. That's why an infant must drink whole milk, and not skim milk.

The following recommendations are intended for those beyond the age of two. The American Heart Association recommends that after the age of two children should share the same healthy diet as adults.

The American Academy of Pediatrics is even more liberal. The AAP feels that teen-agers need red meat, whole milk, and eggs for proper growth and development. The authors disagree — it is in the teen years that eating habits develop which become very hard to change and atherosclerosis begins to form.

Is there an upper age limit? What about grandma, at

age 90? Should she be careful about fat and cholesterol? In the Honolulu Heart Program, they studied elderly men of 65 to 74 years. They found that elevated cholesterol is still a risk factor. It is important to control cholesterol in the young, the middle aged, and the elderly. There is good evidence now that a low-cholesterol diet can reverse atherosclerosis.

The first questions you must ask are: Which members of my family (including myself) are at risk of a myocardial infarction and stroke; and who should alter their life styles?

To answer this question you must know what each member of your family has as risk factors. That is, you must know the blood cholesterol levels, the HDL levels, and the LDL blood levels. Then you must review the chapter on risk.

Of course, it is also important to know about the other risk factors such as smoking, stress, and blood pressure. If you smoke, what you are doing is so destructive that your diet becomes a minor risk factor. So quitting smoking should be your first priority.

The expense of drawing blood cholesterol, triglyceride, and HDL on everyone in the United States is prohibitive. One economical way to screen for lipid abnormalities is for each adult to have blood cholesterol measured every five years. The blood is drawn with the person fasting. If the cholesterol is high, the triglyceride level and HDL are measured. We must be certain that there is no error and that we are seeing a consistently high lipid level. The blood should be redrawn and retested a week or two later. The cholesterol and triglyceride must be measured again before committing someone to long term therapy. In this way we can determine what the major problem is: high cholesterol, high triglyceride, or both. Many experts feel that regardless of expense, the determination of HDL must be measured in everone. A patient with a cholesterol of 180 is still at considerable risk if his HDL is only 25.

If the individual has a high cholesterol but also has a very high HDL, no treatment is needed. On the other hand some people with normal cholesterol should also be measured for HDL, particularly anyone who has had any disease associated with atherosclerosis or has a family history of heart disease.

Hopefully, you are convinced that high cholesterol, high LDL, and low HDL are not good to have in our blood. The next question is, "What can we do about it?"

If you find that your family is at risk, can you really induce them to change their life styles? If you think people are fixed in their ways and no amount of education can cause them to change their eating habits, just study the table below and you will see how wrong you are.

PER CAPITA ANNUAL CONSUMPTION
UNITED STATES

Product	1950	1960	1970	1980	% Change
Eggs(number)	389	334	309	272	-32.9
Milk fat*	29	24	21	20	-27.6
Beef*	63	85	113	103	+68.3
Fish*	12	10	12	13	+16.7
Pork*	69	78	73	73	+ 4.3
Lard*	13	7	5	2	-84.6

*Lbs/person/yr

There have been a few disappointments such as the increased consumption of beef, but in the '80s even that has fallen. In general, people in the United States have greatly decreased their intake of fat. We even have the beef producers worried. Their TV commercials demonstrate that they are running scared. We also see all of these people jogging along streets, dodging the cars. We first became concerned about cholesterol in our diet in the late '60s and early '70s, and as a result there was a 32% decrease in death from heart attacks from 1971 to 1974 and a 49% decrease in the incidence of stroke in the same time.

One reason for this decrease in mortality is that Americans, besides exercising more, are eating more intelligently.

In the chapter Risk we showed how the lipid abnormalities could be divided into nine types. They all had terrible names such as *familial combined hyperlipidemia*. Does that mean each disorder requires a different diet?

Life can be simple at times. The American Heart Association recommends only one diet, to be tried for six months to a year before resorting to drug therapy. It is a three-phase graded program to reduce saturated fat, total fat, and cholesterol. The dieter should follow each phase for at least three weeks before the cholesterol and triglyceride is measured to test the diet's effectiveness.

Forty percent of the average American's daily calories come from fat (with 20% as saturated fat) and 500mg to 600mg of cholesterol. The American Heart Association recommends that the diet be changed as follows:

PHASE I: The diet begins with these alterations: 30% of total calories as fat, 55% as carbohydrate, and 15% as protein. The fat portion should be equal amounts of saturated, monounsaturated, and polyunsaturated fat. Complex carbohydrates should be the major source of total carbohydrates, with less than 300mg of cholesterol eaten each day.

PHASE II: This diet is more strict than that of Phase I. Here, only 25% of calories are fat, again with equal amounts of the three types of fat. The carbohydrate is increased to 60% and the protein remains at 15%. Cholesterol intake is reduced to between 200mg and 250mg each day.

PHASE III: This is the most restricted diet recommended. Only 20% of the calories are fat. The fat is still divided equally among the three types. Cholesterol is restricted to 100 to 150mg each day.

The National Institute of Health recommends a slightly different approach. They advise that all adults undergo a blood cholesterol measurement at least once every five years. People with a cholesterol level greater than 200mg% should adopt a Phase I diet. Those with a cholesterol level above 240 mg% should go to a Phase II diet, and sometimes drugs. With these guidelines, very few of us would escape at least a Phase I diet. Many experts in the field would not encourage strict dietary management until the cholesterol exceeded 240mg%.

Some experts believe that different lipid abnormalities require different diets. The table below summarizes their feelings about diet:

DIET EMPHASIS AND LIPID ABNORMALITY

Abnormality	Caloric Restriction	Decreased Fat & Increased Complex Carbohydrate	Cholesterol Restriction
High cholesterol	+	+++	+++
High triglyceride	+++	+	+
High chol & trig	++	++	++

According to the table above, someone who has a normal cholesterol and high triglycerides should try to loose weight. It is not important for him to watch cholesterol closely. Someone with a high cholesterol, but normal triglycerides does not have to be concerned about decreasing calories, but must reduce cholesterol and fat in the diet.

According to today's literature, the saturated fats seem to be the major culprit. So why not concentrate on reducing the saturated fats alone? Because in a diet restricted to unsaturated fats we commonly find a reduction in HDL. We also see an increase in gallstones.

Actually, monounsaturated fats seem to be as effective as polyunsaturated fats in reducing cholesterol, and cause less of a lowering of HDL. Fish diets lower the incidence of atherosclerosis. There is a direct relationship between the amount of fish consumed in a country and the decrease in heart disease and stroke. We think that this is because of the omega-3 fatty acids found in fish. This family of fatty acids reduce LDL levels, and thereby reduce both blood triglyceride and cholesterol levels. We believe that this occurs because the fish fat inhibits the production of apolipoprotein B which is a component of LDL. In general these are the foods to avoid:

Animal fat	Chocolate
Lunch meats	Ice cream
Hot dogs	Butter
Bacon	Nuts
Organ meats	Whole milk
Beef	Whole milk products
Pork	Saturated oils such as
Caviar	palm, coconut.

That sure takes a lot of joy out of life. What can we eat instead?

Instead of the meats listed in the no-no list:

> Any of the fish with fins and scales are just great. The fish with fins are not only low in cholesterol, but they are high in fish oil, which is good for you. Next would be shellfish, but limit the shellfish to about three ounces per week. You can also substitute poultry for beef, pork, etc., but be sure to remove the skin. Buffalo, believe it or not, is very low in cholesterol and fat.

What about whole milk, ice cream, and all of those other goodies?

> Use skim milk. 1% and 2% milk have too much fat. If you must have ice cream, substitute ice milk or non-fat frozen yogurt. If you must have cheese, there are low-cholesterol cheeses available, such as Muenster, made with skim milk, or low cholesterol Swiss. Other compromises are low-fat cottage cheese, farmer's, hoop, and low-fat ricotta. Remember

that these are compromises. Whether or not you can allow yourself these little liberties depends on the severity of your lipid problem and how easy it is to control.

Fats and oils of all kinds should be limited. In heart disease the saturated fats are the culprit; but there is some data suggesting that breast and bowel cancer is related to total fat intake, and not just the saturated fats. You are obviously going to have to read the labels on your salad dressing bottles and margarine very carefully.

The common polyunsaturated fats are safflower, sunflower, corn, cottonseed, sesame, and soybean oil. When you shop for salad oil, look for the low-calorie salad dressings — these are also the low fat salad dressings. Remember! Carbohydrate and protein have four calories per gram, while fat has a whopping nine calories per gram. You can't have a low-calorie salad dressing that is high in fat.

The monounsaturated oils are also OK, but you are limited to olive and peanut oil.

The saturated fats are the real no-no. Here, we have butter, lard, and cream. Even food labeled as 100% vegetable oil is not safe. The creamers that are used in coffee are loaded with palm or coconut oil, which is very highly saturated.

So you like your eggs. Eggs are very high in cholesterol, but you can get around this.

You can stick to egg whites. There are also cholesterol-free substitutes such as Egg Beaters.

In the table below you will get some additional ideas on how to make healthy substitutions.

HEALTHY SUBSTITUTES

Instead Of This	Eat This
1 cup whipping cream in your cream recipes	3 egg whites with 30 calories and almost no fat
1 cup ice cream with 24 grams fat.	1 cup soy frozen dessert with 5 grams fat
2 tbsp chocolate syrup with 5.5 grams fat	2 tbsp carob syrup with less than 1 gram fat
1/2 cup sour cream with 240 calories and 24 grams fat	1/2 cup low-fat yogurt with 72 calories and 2 grams fat
3 whole eggs with 240 calories and 18 grams fat	3 egg whites with 48 calories and a trace of fat
1 tbsp butter with 14 grams fat	1 tbsp peanut butter with 8 grams fat

What else can you eat? Well, you can eat grains, cereals, and breads, but be careful that coconut or palm oil is not used in the preparation; and you can eat all fruits and vegetables as well as their juices.

You must read labels very carefully. When you see a label that says "Absolutely no cholesterol," should you feel comfortable knowing that that food is safe for your blood vessels. No! Don't trust these people. They will tell you that there is no cholesterol in their mayonnaise-soybean spread, but they don't tell you that it has 1.6 grams of saturated fat in each tablespoon. A popular prominent cereal has .3mg of fiber per ounce. It's a fairly high fiber cereal, but it also contains 4.2 grams of saturated fat per ounce. That makes it a very fatty cereal. The cereal companies are not going to put in big letters on the box, "HIGH IN FAT." Some companies have responded to pressure from the educated consumer. They have stopped using coconut oil and palm oil in their products.

What about the youngsters? It's going to be tough to keep them away from their hot dogs, hamburgers, and French fries, especially while they're away from home, where the influence of their peers is overwhelming. That is why instilling healthy habits by your example is important.

At home you have control over your children's intake of fat. Don't keep whole milk in the house. A cup of whole milk will supply 8.5 grams of fat. A cup of 1% milk cuts this to 2 grams, and skim milk cuts fat even more. Instead of cream cheese, using kefir cheese on sandwiches will cut the fat in half. You can also cut fat in half by substituting soy margarine for butter, vegiburger for hamburger, and tofu mayonnaise for regular mayonnaise. Peanut butter is also a healthy snack, but it's a bit fattening. By substituting two tablespoons carob syrup for the same amount of chocolate syrup, you drop the fat intake from 5.4 grams to 1 gram.

If anyone in your family is overweight, a weight reduction diet is very important. Blood triglyceride drops sharply even when only modest weight is lost. Drugs are often ineffective if the individual remains obese.

We all know how difficult it is to lose weight on a calorie-restricted diet. It becomes easier if diet is combined with exercise, which increases the rate at which we burn fat. You don't need any fancy equipment. A bike, stationary or moving, and/or a nice pair of running shoes will work wonders. There is no diet that will raise HDL significantly, but exercise will.

CALORIES USED PER MINUTE
IN A 150 LB INDIVIDUAL

Running 7.5mph	13 Calories
Swimming 2mph	8- Calories
Bicycling 9.5mph	7 Calories
Walking 3mph	4 Calories
Aerobics	7 Calories

But the benefits are greater than implied by the numbers in the chart. According to the statistics, you must run for twenty minutes to consume about 250 Calories — one slice of chocolate cake. But in addition, we now believe that regular exercise increases your metabolic rate (and therefore your calorie consumption) for the rest of the day.

You only burned 250 calories while running. However, you will continue burning calories at a higher rate even when you are not exercising. The exercise will not only help reduce weight, but will also lower blood cholesterol and raise the HDL. To accomplish this, however, you must exercise a minimum of three days a week for at least twenty minutes at a time. During the exercise period the heart rate must be increased, best accomplished by aerobic type exercise.

In a study conducted on physicians, the long-distant runners were found to have an average HDL of 54mg%. The couch potatoes had an average HDL of only 45mg%. In another study of an even larger population, the couch potatoes had an HDL of 43mg%, the joggers 58mg%, and the marathon runners an average HDL of 65mg%. Lets see how important this is. Suppose that the average cholesterol is 220. What would their ration of cholesterol to HDL be?

couch potato	=	5.1
jogger	=	3.8
marathoners	=	3.4

From the previous chapter, we know that a 5.0 ratio represents the average risk of an American. The jogger and the marathoner have decreased this risk by one half.

What about calorie counting? How much food should I eat each day? Here are
some simple rules to follow.

1. First refer to the table of desirable or ideal weights. Multiply your *ideal* weight by 9 if you are a woman under 45, or by 10 if you are a man or woman over 45. If you are a man under 45, multiply your ideal weight by 11. This number is your basal metabolic caloric need. If you did nothing but sleep all

day, this is the number of calories needed to maintain your ideal weight.

2. To adjust further for age, subtract 10 calories for each year over age 25.

3. To adjust for activity, multiply the above number by the following factors:

   x 1.3 if sedentary (office work or couch potato)

   x 1.4 if you occasionally exercise

   x 1.5 if you have a regular exercise program

   x 2 if you are into competitive sports

If you were a 50-year-old man who should weigh 180 pounds, you would have the following basal metabolic need: 180 x 10 - (10 x25) = 1550. You also go to the gym four times a week. You need 1550 x 1.5, or 2325 calories. If you happened to weigh 210 pounds but your ideal weight was 180 pounds at that activity level, you still would need 2325 calories.

The chapters on recipes showed you how food in a low-cholesterol life style can be tasty, and not boring. There is also an appendix listing many foods with their fat content and their cholesterol content.

Another factor to consider is the medications we take for problems that may be unrelated to our lipids. This and the various drugs used to control cholesterol when all else fails are covered in the chapter on pharmacology. It will discusses the control of lipids after you have found that weight control, diet, and exercise did not bring your lipids to acceptable levels. And if you want to know what tobacco, alcohol, and steroids are doing to your lipids, you'll find out in the same chapter.

Obviously you must have guidance from your physician when you undertake control of your blood lipids. There is a major problem here, however. Many physicians are poorly informed about the importance of cholesterol. We tend to treat disease after the fact.

Preventive medicine has only recently become of major concern. A few years ago we discovered how devastating high blood pressure can be to the body. It took a long educational process to convince doctors that they should give pills to people who felt entirely well. They had to give these medicines knowing that the patients would suffer the side effects. Convincing physicians that it was better for the patient to feel ill from side effects than to feel well and have high blood pressure was difficult.

With modern drugs we are lucky. We now can find medications that have minimal side effects, but we have had some bad years. About 1000 charts were reviewed at the Family Health Center at the University of California. Only 33% of the charts had any mention of the patients' cholesterol. Of patients with elevated cholesterol, only 34% were treated.

Now we are more aware that high cholesterol limits life expectancy. We must convince physicians that it is important for patients to take expensive pills. The pills lower the cholesterol but don't make the patient feel better. Some side effects may even make the patient feel worse. It seems logical that anyone who is found to have coronary artery disease should have their cholesterol checked. Certainly the lipids should be checked before the patient goes for a heart catheterization.

Dr. Watt, a physician who does heart catheterizations, published his experience in the journal *Heart Lung*. He found that half the patients sent to him for heart catheterization had elevated cholesterol. Nearly half of those patients did not know they had abnormal lipids before coming to catheterization. Those doctors obviously need to be educated about the importance of measuring serum lipids in their patients.

So, what have we learned in this chapter? Our children must learn by our example. We must teach them to read food labels, and be concerned about what they eat and how they exercise. We can control our cholesterol by maintaining proper body weight, by reducing our intake of saturated fats, and by exercise. All of these variables are inter-related. By cutting fat we cut calories. Exercise also helps us reduce weight, but even if there is no weight change, exercise will lower our cholesterol. Exercise will also raise the high density lipoproteins (HDL). HDL is a potent protector against atherosclerosis. Only when exercise and strict diet fail do we move on to drug therapy.

Chapter IX

PILLS AND THEIR ILLS

OK, so you had a cholesterol of 400mg% and a HDL of only 30. You have restricted your diet by following Phase III for six months, and you run six miles four days a week. Your cholesterol is down to 300mg% and your HDL has risen to 40. You have decreased your cholesterol by 25%, and your cholesterol to HDL ratio has dropped from 13.3 to 7.2.

That's quite an improvement, but it still leaves you in a high risk category. In fact, your risk of getting a heart attack is about double that of the average person. Diet and exercise must be continued, but drugs have to be added.

There are many drugs now available. When any disease has several drugs for its treatment, it tells you something. It tells you that none of the drugs is perfect, otherwise its competitors would be gone from the market.

Below are the recommendations that were widely accepted in 1985. With the information we receive almost daily, there have not only been changes in the recommendations, but many areas of disagreement.

Antihyperlipemics

Lipoprotein Elevation	Drugs of 1st Choice	Drugs of 2nd Choice
Chylomicrons	None	None
Chylomicrons+IDL	Atromid-S	Nicotinic acid
LDL	Cholestyramine	Lorelco, choloxin
VLDL	Nicotinic acid Lopid	Atromid-S
VLDL+LDL	Nicotinic acid Lopid	Atromid-S Cholestyramine

Let's discuss each drug individually. You will see that each has its advantages and disadvantages, and the choice is never simple.

BILE ACID BINDING RESINS: The generic names for this class are colestipol and cholestyramine; The brand names are *Colestipol*, and *Questran*. These drugs are really absorbing resins, and they are not absorbed from the gastrointestinal tract into the circulation. They bind and trap bile acids that pass from the gall bladder into the intestine. Without the drugs, these bile acids, which are made from cholesterol, are reabsorbed through the gut wall and end up back in the circulation. However, once they are trapped by the resin they pass into the stool. The effect, however, is only to lower the LDL in the blood. Triglycerides are not lowered, and may actually rise.

Major side effects: Constipation and bloating are the major problems. Often the problem of constipation can be overcome by increasing the amount of fiber in the diet. Eating oat bran with plenty of fluids will not only soften the stool, but it will aide in lowering the cholesterol. Some patients will get diarrhea, however. Another major problem is that these resins may bind other medications that you are taking, and your physician may have to increase the dose to compensate. An important example is the anticoagulant coumadin. A major problem is that these drugs may raise triglycerides and therefore should not be used in people with hypertriglyceridemia.

Dose: Colestipol comes in 5 gram packages. You begin with one package three times a day, and if needed, slowly increase to two packages three times a day. Cholesteramine comes in 4 gram packages, with a maximum dose of eight packages each day.

Uses: Best to use these drugs to lower LDL. If VLDL and/or hypertriglyceridemia is a problem, other drugs must be added.

NICOTINIC ACID: This is good old niacin. You don't even need a prescription for it because it's a vitamin. Please note, nicotinamide will not work. This drug inhibits the secretion of VLDL and thereby lowers the concentration of LDL which is formed from VLDL. The breakdown of HDL is decreased by nicotinic acid, and as a result you will see a rise in HDL.

Common side effects: Flushing is a common but harmless side effect. It is caused by dilatation of the blood vessels in the skin. The flushing can be blunted by taking one aspirin tablet about thirty minutes before the niacin. Rash and itching is also common. Liver function blood tests must be done periodically. If the niacin is taken with a resin, these problems are rarely encountered. People with stomach ulcers should avoid the drug. If you have a history of gout, nicotinic acid might cause a new attack. It may also cause an abnormality in the liver in some people.

Dosage: How can a vitamin have so many side effects? It is because it is not taken as a vitamin. The daily requirement of niacin is about 20mg. If you are taking it to control blood lipids you start at 100mg three times each day with a maximum dose of 7500mg each day. These are not vitamin doses, but are pharmacological doses. Even though you can get this drug without a prescription, it should not be taken in these amounts without the close guidance of a physician. Niacin is sold in these doses as Nicolar, which comes in 500mg tablets. If you took 20mg niacin tablets, you would have to take twenty-five tablets to get the equivalent of one Nicolar.

Uses: With a resin, niacin commonly brings LDL to normal levels.

CLOFIBRATE: Also known by its brand name *Atromid-S*. The major effect is to lower VLDL. This drug increases the activity of an enzyme that breaks down triglyceride rich lipoproteins. This sounds like a good thing, but the breakdown products of these lipoproteins go into the manufacturing of LDL. So, in a patient with hypertriglyceridemia, this drug may increase LDL.

Major side effects: Nausea and abdominal discomfort are the major complaints. The major problem is a 200% to 400% increase in the incidence of gall stones. There may also be a slight increase in gastrointestinal cancer. Other problems are baldness, loss of sex drive, liver toxicity, and a decrease in the ability of the bone marrow to make blood.

Dose: 250mg to 1000mg twice each day.

Uses: For the reduction of triglyceride-rich lipoproteins in diseases such as those with very high levels of chylomicrons or VLDL.

GEMFIBROZIL: This is one of the newest agents available, and it is marketed as *Lopid*. It closely resembles clofibrate in its action, but it not only lowers VLDL, but also raises HDL. It also lowers LDL. In a five-year study, about 2000 men were given *Lopid*, while another group of more than 2000 were given a placebo. In the *Lopid* group, 27% developed heart problems during the study. In the placebo group, 41% had heart disease develop.

Major side effects: Like *Atromid-S* it may cause gastrointestinal side effects. Tests for liver and bone marrow function must also be done. It should not be used with lovastatin.

Dose: Usually 600mg twice each day.

Uses: Used for the same conditions appropriate for *Atromid-S,* but probably much more effective and safer.

PROBUCOL: The brand name for this drug is *Lorelco.* It is thought to lower LDL level in the blood by combining with it, forming a larger particle that is more rapidly removed from the blood. One very serious drawback back is that it lowers HDL more than it lowers LDL. Probucol also prevents the deposition of LDL on arterial walls. HDL commonly reaches levels of 10mg% or less.

Common side effects: Nausea, diarrhea and abdominal pain.

Dose: 500mg twice each day.

Uses: In spite of the worrisome fact that it lowers HDL, treatment with this drug results in disappearance of cholesterol plaques in the skin.

DEXTROTHYROXIN: The molecule of this drug is the mirror image of that of thyroid. But to the body, there is a great deal of differences in properties between substances that are are mirror images. This drug is sold under the brand name of *Choloxin.* It retains some of the properties of Levothyroxin or thyroid. It increases the conversion of LDL to bile, and thereby decreases the level of LDL in the blood.

Common side effects: Unfortunately, the drug has some thyroid-effect on the body, although to a much lesser degree than thyroid itself. Thyroid is similar to the idle control in your car's carburetor. Thyroid increases metabolic rate. It makes your heart beat faster and work harder. Someone with heart disease may have problems with angina or abnormal heart rhythms when taking this drug.

Dosage: 4mg to 8mg each day.

Uses: This drug reduces serum cholesterol only by 20%, and therefore should be used to treat only mild elevations of cholesterol. The individual taking this medication should have no signs or symptoms of heart disease, and have been found not to tolerate other cholesterol-lowering medications.

LOVASTATIN: This is a new drug marketed as *Mevacor*. It actually decreases the rate of manufacturing cholesterol, by interfering with the action of an enzyme (a catalyst) that the body uses for building cholesterol molecules. It is a remarkably effective medication.

Major side effects: This drug would probably replace all the other cholesterol-lowering drugs, if it weren't for some major problems. It will occasionally cause abnormal liver chemistries, so people on this drug require frequent blood testing. We must also recommend that the patient be seen by an ophthalmologist. Eye problems have also been associated with this drug. Both of these factors add extra expense to an already expensive medication.

Use: A very effective cholesterol-lowering agent, but safer drugs should probably be tried first.

Dose: One to four tablets each day.

DRUG COMBINATIONS: There are certain circumstances when two or more drugs must be used. One drug may not lower the serum cholesterol to a desirable range. If both LDL and VLDL are elevated two drugs may be needed. Occasionally there is an increase in VLDL when a resin is used to treat an elevated LDL, and another drug must be added.

Oat bran and psyllium have also been found to be effective in lowering cholesterol.Psyllium has been found in bulking agents such as Metamucil. Although they may not be quite as effective as some of our prescription medications, they are also not quite as expensive. Some experts feel that bran works by merely replacing other foods, and does not have a direct effect on your cholersterol. After you have a cup of bran you are too full to eat your steak. Regardless of their mechanism of action, by using these inexpensive substances together with a careful diet, your physician may be able to lower your dose of the more expensive prescription medications.

Guar gum has also been studied for its effects on lipids. Eating crackers made of quar gum dropped the LDL cholesterol by 13%. There were problems with the gum sticking to the roof of the mouth and the production of an excess of intestinal gas. This method of cholesterol reduction holds promise, but needs much improvement.

We must be very careful using over-the-counter drugs that have not been fully proven. We know from reading a previous chapter that fish is good for you. The higher the fish consumption in a given country, the lower the incidence of atherosclerosis. Since this is probably due to certain oils in the fish, why not skip the fish itself and just drink the oil? The oils are generally available over the counter under various brand names such as *MaxEPA*, and logically should be beneficial.

The beneficial oils found in fish are called omega-3 fatty acids. Fatty acids are made up of carbon atoms strung in a chain. On one end is an organic acid, and the rest of the carbon atoms are loaded with hydrogen atoms. If two hydrogen atoms are missing, you have an unsaturated fatty acid. An omega-3 fatty acid is unsaturated, counting 3 carbon atoms from the end not having the acid part.

LINOLENIC ACID

```
   H   H   H   H   H   H   H   H   H   H   H   H   H   H   H   H   H  O -H
   |   |   |   |   |   |   |   |   |   |   |   |   |   |   |   |   |  |
H -C - C - C =C - C - C = C - C - C= C - C - C - C - C - C - C - C - C =O
   |   |           |           |           |   |   |   |   |   |   |
   H   H           H           H           H   H   H   H   H   H   H
   1   2   3   4   5   6   7   8   9   10  11  12  13  14  15  16  17  18
```

This is called Linolenic acid. It is 18 carbon atoms long and is unsaturated at carbon positions 3,6, and 9. Because the first place that it is unsaturated is position 3, it is called a 3-omega acid. This fatty acid is found in marine algae, plankton, and fish. In 1975, Eskimos were found to have a much lower LDL and a much higher HDL in comparison to Danes. Experiments on primates and humans have shown that feeding of fish oil decreases the synthesis of cholesterol by the liver. There is also the production of smaller particles of LDL. Small LDL has less cholesterol, less big LDL, and causes less atherosclerosis. If total LDL is measured, no significant change may be seen in LDL. However, people who consume fish oil have the small LDL and are less likely to develop atherosclerosis.

Fatty acids are used in the construction of membranes of cells. An increase in the unsaturated fatty acids in the membranes results in a decrease in the amount of saturated fatty acids. In order for atherosclerosis to form in a blood vessel, the vessel wall must be damaged. Perhaps cell membranes constructed using fish oils are less likely to be damaged, and thus decreasing chances for atherosclerosis.

Omega-3 acids also reduce the production of various potent vasoconstrictors by the body. These vasoconstrictors cause blood vessels to constrict and platelets to form clots, so they may rob tissue of blood flow and make tissue susceptible to atherosclerosis. The formation of clots also rob tissue of blood supply and is one of the major mechanisms of creating myocardial infarctions.

Omega-3 fatty acids also make the blood less viscous. When the blood is more fluid, it can pass more easily through narrow blood vessels. Not only do these fatty acids prevent the formation of clots, but they tend do cause the dissolving of clots already formed. Omega-3 acids also reduce triglyceride production.

To summarize all of these effects, omega-3 fatty acids:

1. Inhibits vasoconstriction (the narrowing of blood vessels by contraction of muscle in the vessel wall)

2. Reduce clumping of platelets and clot formation

3. Stimulate the dissolution of clots

4. Make blood less viscous and more fluid

5. Reduce blood pressure

6. Raise HDL and lower LDL in some people

7. Lower cholesterol and triglycerides

8. Make smaller and less atherogenic LDL

What about human studies regarding the incidence of myocardial infarction? The following table compares three populations, each having different amounts of omega-6 and omega-3 acids in their blood. This is related to death rate.

	Ratio omega-6 to omega-3	Coronary Disease (% death)
Europe, USA	50	40
Japan	12	12
Greenland Eskimo	1.2	7

Epidemiological studies have shown that eating just thirty-five grams (a bit more than one ounce) of fish each day will reduce mortality from atherosclerosis by fifty percent.

Ok! Fish oil sounds great. How much should I feed to my family? No good data exists to answer this question. Remember, the Eskimos have been eating fish for a lifetime. We may have been spending more than half of our life eating the wrong food. How much fish oil do we have to eat to catch up with the eskimos? The most commonly available preparations are capsules containing 0.3 grams of omega-3 fatty acid. In many clinical studies, four grams of omega-3 oil was given each day. So, you would have to take about thirteen capsules each day. This much omega-3 oil tends to cause nausea.

Cod liver oil is not very helpful. Although it has 20%

omega-3, it also has large amounts of vitamins A and D. Vitamins A and D are toxic when taken in large amounts. This limits the amount you can safely drink. Physicians are not ready to prescribe omega-3 capsules to the public.

Not all seafood is rich in omega-3 fatty acids. The oily fish such as mackerel, lake trout, herring, sardine, tuna and salmon, have 1.5 to 2.6 grams of omega-3 fatty acid per 100 grams of edible fish. On the other hand, lobster, cod, shrimp, crab, and oyster have less than one gram of this fat per 100 grams of meat.

Are there any problems with a diet rich in fish? With the fish comes the pollution from our rivers and lakes. The chlorinated hydrocarbons are known to cause cancer, and the mercury is known to destroy the brain. The tendency to bleed may be slightly increased with a fish diet, but this does not seem to be clinically significant.

Not all scientific studies have supported these findings regarding fish oil. In one study, volunteers were given encapsulated fish oil, resulting in a rise in cholesterol of 14% and a rise in HDL of 13%. The ratio of cholesterol to HDL was increased. There was a fall in triglyceride level, but this was not significant. Therefore, in this study it appears that fish oil supplements may have had an adverse effect on lipids.

At the University of Kentucky, there have been several studies to see how well oat bran lowers cholesterol. People on diets containing about 100 grams of oat bran each day had a decrease of 19% in cholesterol and no reduction in HDL. The oat bran was added to an average American diet, and no attempt was made to reduce the saturated fat in the diet. How does it work? One theory is that the oat fibers bind bile acids so they cannot be reabsorbed. As a result, the liver is forced to manufacture new bile acid from its supply of cholesterol. In this way the body's supply of cholesterol is depleted.

What about alcohol? Alcohol in moderation appears to give some protection from coronary artery disease. It probably does this by increasing the concentrations of some of the HDL subfractions. Alcohol also raises blood pressure, destroys the stomach, brain and liver, and can cause a disease of the heart muscle called "alcoholic cardiomyopathy." But alcoholics don't seem to have as many heart attacks as the rest of the population. When a group of volunteers were given one beer each day for eight weeks, they had a rise in apolipoprotein A1. Apolipoprotein A1 is an important component of both triglycerides and HDL. The rise in this apolipoprotein protects from atherosclerosis. I don't think we can recommend alcohol to control lipids.

Besides genetic predisposition and diet, other factors must be considered. What medications are you taking? If you are into body building and you're sneaking steroids such as testosterone, you can figure on a marked reduction in HDL. The common drugs that reduce HDL are;

steroids such as testosterone

steroids such as cholesterol

steroids such as provera

probucol(lorelco)

tobacco

That's right! The next to the last drug, probucol, lowers cholesterol by lowering LDL. Unfortunately, it also lowers HDL. Remember, HDL is the "good" cholesterol fraction. This effect on HDL may make it seem to be less than an ideal drug for hyperlipidemia. If lorelco has an adverse effect on HDL, why is it used? The fact remains, lorelco has been shown to decrease the size of cholesterol deposits in several studies. The drug works in spite of its theoretical limitations.

School age children who start smoking have a drop in HDL within two years. Smoking one pack of cigarettes a day caused a drop of 8mg% of HDL. This greatly increases the risk of atherosclerosis. The damage done during these early years starts a vascular process that may continue even after smoking stops.

There are also some drugs that we use for high blood pressure that have an effect on lipids.

EFFECT OF ANTIHYPERTENSIVE DRUGS ON LIPID

Drug	Lipid Effect
Diuretics(hydrochloro-thiazide, zaroxolyn, lasix)	Adverse
Beta-blockers(inderal, corgard, tenormin, lopressor)	Adverse
ISA Beta-blockers(acebutolol, atenolol)	Neutral
Alpha-blockers(minipress)	Favorable
Alpha+Beta-blocker(labetalol)	Favorable
Aldomet	Neutral
ACE inhibitors(capoten, zestril, vasotec)	Neutral

Drug	Lipid Effect
Calcium channel blockers(procardia, verapamil, cardizem)	Neutral

We do not have space to include all members of a particular class in each category. Many drugs have not been tested. If you are taking a particular drug, as a diuretic for instance, it is safe to assume that it shares the other diuretic's adverse properties toward lipids. Not everyone's studies agree. Several researchers have found that diuretics increase LDL cholesterol, yet in one study, they found the effect on lipids was negligible. Not all diuretics share this property regarding lipids. Lozol has no effect on lipids. Note that not all beta blockers are alike. Some have an adverse effect on lipids, and some a favorable effect. Propranolol(inderal) raises triglyceride levels, while oxprenalol raises HDL. Recently it was discovered that patients treated with Inderal had an acceleration in the progression of atherosclerosis as compared with patients treated with Pocardia. However, the lives saved by the control of blood pressure with Inderal greatly exceeds the number of lives lost due to adverse effects on lipids. Don't stop you Inderal. Remember, there are other properties of drugs besides their effect on lipid levels. Your physician may feel that these other properties give such an advantage that you must compromise and use a drug that raises cholesterol or lowers HDL. As an example, lopressor belongs to that group of beta-blockers that raises cholesterol. But if you have had a heart attack, or are at risk of having a heart attack, you are much less likely to get that heart attack, if you take lopressor.

There are many other medications besides antihypertensives that effect lipids. Information is scattered. Only recently has there been enough interest to warrant such studies. In the following table are listed three other commonly used drugs. Two are used to treat patients with stomach ulcers, and one is used to treat dangerous heart rhythms.

LIPID EFFECTS OF VARIOUS DRUGS

Medication	Common Use	Lipid Effect
Tagamet	peptic ulcer disease	raises HDL 30%
Zantac	peptic ulcer disease	no effect
Amiodarone	heart rhythm	raises chol & trig

There are also some common diseases, such as diabetes, hypothyroidism, nephrotic syndrome, uremia, cirrhosis, and alcoholism that are associated with lipid abnormalities. To treat the lipid abnormality effectively, you must first treat the underlying disease.

There is a lot of information stuffed into this chapter. The table below is a summary of the properties of many of the lipid-lowering agents that we use. Under the heading of cholesterol is listed the percent reduction that would be expected for each agent. Under the heading of triglycerides are listed pluses and minuses. The more pluses seen, the greater the expected reduction in triglyceride.

Agent	Cost/day To Pharmacist	Efficacy In Reducing Cholesterol	Trig
Lorelco	$1.41	11 to 27%	++
Questran	$2.50 (bulk powd)	13 to 25%	0

Colestid	$3.05 (granules)	13 to 25%	0
Mevacor	$1.56 to $6.25	18 to 34%	++
Nicolar	$1.78 to $3.56	9.6%	+++
Atromid-S	$1.28	6.5 to 9%	+++
Lopid	$1.39	1.8 to 8.6%	+++

Other costs are not obvious from this table. If you use *Mevacor*, for example, you should include the cost of having your eyes examined by an ophthalmologist. Occasional blood tests are also required.

Many new drugs are on the horizon. These medications must be fully investigated. When their safety is established, they will then be given limited and very controlled trials in humans.

The following is a listing of some of these agents. Some will be available by the time this book is published, some are years away from release, and some will be found to turn skin green and cause hair to fall out. Here are some of the drugs you may be hearing about in the future:

Etofibrate   Simavastatin   Bezafibrate

Mevinolin   Acarbose

What about the person who doesn't respond to any of the medications but continues to have dangerously abnormal lipids? Other techniques are being tried to lower lipids:

Partial Ileal Bipass: A surgeon opens the abdomen, cuts the small bowel, and rearranges the pipes. The contents of the stomach pass through only a portion of the small intestine before entering the large intestine. Because of this short-cut, the lipid absorption that would occur in the ilium is avoided. Another drastic technique is to pass the patient's blood through a device that filters out the lipids, and then the blood is returned to the patient. Of course this has to be repeated on a regular basis to be effective. The number of drugs available is steadily increasing. No single drug is the total answer. Drugs should be used only when exercise and diet fails. When a drug is started, the diet and exercise should continue. In this way we can keep the dose of the medication to a minimum, and thereby minimize the chance of side effects.

Chapter X

JUST ONE MORE LITTLE WORD

After a meal, you're often tempted by "one little mint." So we'd like to tempt you into reading just a few more words.

As far as the recipes are concerned, we have to admit that we are not trained chefs. We enjoy food. We look with pleasure at a nicely set table surrounded by family and friends.

As physicians and caring human beings, we know which foods are wholesome. And, of course, we know what tastes good to us. We've put all that together in our recipes.

The recipes are really there to give you a feel for meals that are kind to your arteries. They're starting points for you to teach your children. Your youngsters will see that food can be low in cholesterol, yet attractive and delicious.

Many of your favorite recipes can be made the low-cholesterol way, with no loss of taste. Through the years, we have experimented with making our old cherished recipes healthier. For example, recipes with baked bananas instruct you to add margarine or butter. We add no oil and don't notice any difference in flavor.

When you experiment, you'll certainly have cooking disasters. This is the way you learn. And those disasters make great dinner-time stories!

Don't be uneasy when you find your child tearing into a bag of greasy potato chips. You know yourself that there are times when nothing but a hot dog will satisfy you at the game.

Just don't put a lot of emphasis on a lack of perfection in food choices. As everybody says, "We're only human."

Gently, through your life style, let your young ones know that fruit, oat bran muffins, and unbuttered pop corn are flavorful. Be sure plenty of the good stuff is available to them. And when they have two pieces of that whipped cream layered birthday cake, it's OK. It's like a formal gown or tuxedo. You certainly don't wear it all the time. Now and then, it's a lot of fun.

Keep in mind that if you're eating healthfully at least eighty percent of the time, you're doing very well indeed.

Make a healthy life style a family affair. You can do that by shopping and preparing meals together.

Exercise is also something we do as a family unit. Take bicycle rides together. Plan a rest stop and enjoy packable fruits and vegetables.

If someone in your family can't ride a bike, there's nothing like a brisk walk around the neighborhood. Exercise is simply physical activity. You don't have to spend hours on Nautilus equipment or train for a triathlon to reap its benefits.

Using meal planning, shopping, and exercise as object lessons and instruction for your children will make them aware of the low-cholesterol lifestyle. This brings the family closer, as you interact in discussions about what you have learned and would like to try.

There's a lot of information out there. Magazines, family sections of the newspaper, and books (like this one). All of us are learning continuously.

So, happy, healthy, and joyous eating from our family to yours.

GLOSSARY

Angina: Means choking. A discomfort felt, usually in the chest, caused by inadequate blood flow through the coronary arteries that feed the heart muscle.

Apoprotein: A protein that is commonly attached to a lipid.

Arteriosclerosis: A thickening and hardening of the walls of the arteries.

Atheroma: A fatty deposit on the walls of arteries.

Atherosclerosis: Arteriosclerosis where the deposition of lipid is in clumps. Atherosclerosis and arteriosclerosis are used interchangeably by many authors.

Centrifuge: A machine that spins material at very high speed, so that heavier or more dense material moves the furthest from the center of spin. In this way substance can be separated from each other according to their density.

Cholesterol: A lipid whose molecule is a complex ring structure. It is found in many parts of the animal including atheromatous plaques and gallstones, but also a necessary part of the brain and many hormones.

Coronary artery: The arteries that supply blood to heart muscle. When the flow of blood through these arteries are partially obstructed you get angina and when totally obstructed you get death of heart muscle (a myocardial infarction).

Double blind study: Testing in which neither the researcher or the subject know whether or not they are getting the real drug or the placebo. See Placebo.

Fat: A substance made up of lipids.

High density lipoprotein: A fatty protein that falls to the bottom when serum is spun in an ultracentrifuge.

HDL: High density lipoprotein.

Lipid: A fatty substance soluble in organic solvents such as oils rather than water.

Lipoprotein: A molecule that consists of a lipid attached to a protein.

LDL: Low density lipoprotein. A lipoprotein that comes to the top of the tube and rests just below the VLDL when serum is spun in an ultracentrifuge.

Milligrams percent(mg%): A measure of concentration commonly used in medicine. It means the number of milligrams of a substance dissolved in 100ml (or cc) of blood or other body fluid.

Myocardial Infarction: *Myocardial* means heart muscle and *infarction* means death of tissue. The lay term for myocardial infarction is heart attack.

Placebo: A so-called sugar pill. When we study the effectiveness of new drugs it is common to give half the patients fake pills. Neither the patient or the doctors should know who is getting the fake pills. In this way the results of the tests are unbiased.

Plaque: A fatty build-up on the wall of an artery. It is made up of various breakdown products of blood. A major component of a plaque is cholesterol.

Saturated fat: A fat in which all places on the molecule that can hold hydrogen atoms do hold hydrogen atoms. The molecule is "saturated" with hydrogen.

Stroke: A lay term that denotes a cerebrovascular accident. This is death of brain tissue either from an obstruction of blood flow to the brain or hemorrhage into the brain.

Unsaturated fat: There is at least one area on the molecule of fat (a double bond) where a hydrogen molecule can be added. Monounsaturated means that there is one such position, and polyunsaturated means that there is more than one such position.

Very Low Density Lipoprotein: A lipoprotein that tends to float to the very top when serum is spun in an ultracentrifuge. The lightest of the lipoprotein molecules.

Ultracentrifuge: A very high speed centrifuge.

Xanthomas: Fatty deposits in the skin.

REFERENCES

We are being drowned in the scientific literature about lipids. In August of 1988 alone, there were about thirty-five important original research papers with lipids as their topic. Below are listed only a few that are of interest. If you have any doubt of the validity of the advice given in this book, we encourage you to read the literature.

The chart in this book on the nutrient content of food is only a small fraction of the data extracted from the reference below:

Pennington J, Church H: *Food Values*, 14th Ed Harper & Row, New York.

For those who wish to evaluate their own recipes, I highly recommend:

Jacobson, M: "Nutrition Wizard", Center for Science in the Public Interest, 1501 16th Street, N.W., Washington, D.C. 20036, 202/332-9110. This is an inexpensive program that will calculate the nutrient content of your recipes. Very simple and powerful.

The technically minded will find the following references to be excellent sources to expand their knowlege.

Anderson J, Zettwock N, et al: "Cholesterol-Lowering Effects of Psyllium Hydrophilic Mucilloid for Hypercholesterolemic Men." *Arch Intern Med* 1988;148:292-296.

Arkey R, Perlman A: "Scientific American Medicine Hyper lipoproteinemia", *Scientific American*, 1988, ch 9.2, pp 1-9.

Dwyer J, Rieger-Ndakorerwa G, et al: "Low-Level Cigarette Smoking and Longitudinal Change in Serum Cholesterol Among Adolescents: The Berlin-Bremen Study." *JAMA* 1988;259:2857-2862.

Gordon T, Sorlie P, Kannel WB: *Coronary Heart Disease, Atherothrombotic Brain Infarction, Intermittent Claudication - A Multivariate Analysis of Some Factors Related to Their Incidence: Framingham study, 16-Year Followup.* Section 27, Government Printing Office, 1971.

Hoegg JM, Gregg RE, Brewer HB Jr: "An approach to the management of hyperlipoproteinemia." *JAMA* 1986;255:512-521.

Kannel W, Castelli W, et al: "Serum cholesterol, lipoproteins, and risk of coronary heart disease: The Framingham study." *Ann Intern Med* 1971;74:1-12.

Lipid Research Clinics Program: "The Lipid Research Clinics Coronary Primary Prevention Trial results: I. Reduction in incidence of coronary heart disease." *JAMA* 1984;251:351-64.

Parmley, William and Chatterjee. *Cardiology.* Philadelphia: J. B. Lippincott Co, 1989.

Report of the National Cholesterol Education Program Expert Panel on detection, evaluation and treatment of high cholesterol in adults. *Arch Intern Med* 1988;148:36-69.

Scientific American Medicine. New York: Scientific American, 1989.

Schuler G, Schlierf G, et al: "Low-Fat Diet and Regular, Supervised Physical Exercise in Patients With Symptomatic Coronary Artery Disease: Reduction of Stress-Induced Myocardial Ischemia." *Circulation* 1988;77:172-181.

Superko H, Haskell W, et al: "Effects of Solid and Liquid Guar Gum on Plasma Cholesterol and Triglyceride Concentrations in Moderate Hypercholesterolemia." *Am J Cardiol* 1988;62:51-55.

FOOD VALUES

This table is extracted from *Food Values* by Pennington & Church. You will notice that some places on the table are blank. Unfortunately, we don't have complete information on all the foods listed. Please don't assume that a blank means zero. At the saturated fat position for Arby's roast beef sandwich there is a blank. I can asure you that there is more than zero grams of saturated fat in their sandwich.

	K Cal	Total Fat (g)	Poly-Uns. Fat (g)	Sat. Fat (g)	Chol (mg)	Fiber (g)
BEVERAGES, CREAMS, ETC						
Apple juice 6oz	92	0.0				
Beer 4.5%alc 12oz	148	0.0				
Beer, light 12oz	100	0.0				
Buttermilk 8oz	99	2.2	0.0	1.3	9	
Coffee 6oz	3	0.0				
Cool whip, 1Tbsp	13	1.0	0.0	1.0	0.0	0.0
Cream, sour 1Tbsp	26	2.5	0.0	1.6	5.0	0.0
Cream, whipping 1Tbsp	52	5.6	0.2	3.5	21.0	0.0

	K Cal	Total Fat (g)	Poly-Uns. Fat (g)	Sat. Fat (g)	Chol (mg)	Fiber (g)
Eggnog 4oz	335	15.8				
Gatorade 8oz	39	0.0				
Grape juice 6oz	89	0.0				
Half & Half, 1Tbsp	20	1.7	0.0	1.1	6.0	0.0
Ice cream, choc 1cup	295	16.0				
Ice cream, van 1cup	269	14.3	0.5	8.9	59.0	0.0
Lemonade 12oz	138	0.0				
Milk, 1% 8oz	119	2.9	0.1	1.8	10	
Milk, 2% 8oz	121	4.7	0.2	2.9	18	
Milk, human 8oz	168	9.2	1.6	4.8	32	
Milk, skim 8oz	86	0.4	0.0	0.3	4	
Milk, soy 8oz	87	4.0			0	
Milk, whole 8oz	150	8.0	0.2	4.9	34	
Milkshake, 1 av choc	356	8.1	0.3	5.0	32	0.8
Orange juice 6oz	92	0.0				
Pepsi cola 12oz	156	0.0				
Pet, powd crm subs 1teas	10	1.0				
Red wine 3.5oz	76	0.0				
Seven-up 12oz	144	0.0				
Tea 8oz	0	0.0				
White wine 3.5oz	80	0.0				
Yogurt, low fat 8oz	144	3.5	0.1	2.3	14	
Yogurt, whole milk 8oz	139	7.4	0.4	4.8	29.0	

CANDY, CAKE & PIE

	K Cal	Total Fat (g)	Poly-Uns. Fat (g)	Sat. Fat (g)	Chol (mg)	Fiber (g)
Almond Joy, 1oz	151	7.8				
Angel food cake, 1pce	161	0.1				
Apple 1/8pie	282	11.9				0.5
Apple streusel, 1pce	200	8.3				0.3
Black forest, 1/8cake	194	9.3				0.3

	K Cal	Total Fat (g)	Poly- Uns. Fat (g)	Sat. Fat (g)	Chol (mg)	Fiber (g)
Boston cream pie, 1/8cake	260	8.0			20	
Butter pecan, 1/12cake	250	11.0				
Carmels, 3 pieces	112	2.9				0.1
Carrot, 1/12cake	250	11.0				
Cheesecake, 1/6cake	300	14.3	1.1	8.9	30	0.1
Choc brownie, 1pce	130	5.0				
Choc chips, milk choc 2oz	218	11.0			7.1	
Choc devils food, 1pce	191	9.3				0.2
Choc fudge, 1 piece	129	4.8				0.1
Choc, Hershey dark 1oz	157	8.6	0.0	6.0	0	0.3
Choc, milk Hershey 1oz	160	9.4	1.0	7.0	10	0.3
Coconut, 1/8cake	246	13.1				0.7
Custard pie, 1pce	327	16.6				
Fruitcake, dark 1pce	152	6.1				0.2
Jelly beans, 10 pieces	66	0.0				
Kit kat, 1.5oz	210	11.0				0.1
Life savers, 5 pieces	39	0.1				
Marble, 1/12cake	270	11.0				
Milky Way, 2.1oz	260	9.0				
Mr. Goodbar, 2oz	300	18.0	3.2	9.5	8	0.6
Peanut butter cups, 2	184	10.7	3.0	6.0	5	0.3
Pound, 1pce	123	5.6				
Shortcake, 1pce	86	2.0				
Sponge, 1pce	113	4.2				0.1

CEREALS, COOKED

Barley, pearled 1/4cup	172	0.5				0.5
Buckwheat groats, 1oz	98					

	K Cal	Total Fat (g)	Poly-Uns. Fat (g)	Sat. Fat (g)	Chol (mg)	Fiber (g)
Corn grits, inst 1pkt	82	0.2				0.1
Cream of Wheat, 3/4cup	100	0.4				
Oats, inst 1pkt	104	1.7			0	0.3

CEREALS, READY TO EAT

	K Cal	Total Fat (g)	Poly-Uns. Fat (g)	Sat. Fat (g)	Chol (mg)	Fiber (g)
All Bran, 1oz(1/3cup)	71	0.5				2.0
Alpen, 1oz	110	5.0				
Bran, 100% 1oz	76	1.4	0.8	0.3		2.1
Bran Flakes, 40% 1oz	93	0.5				1.0
Cap'n Crunch, 1oz	119	2.6	0.4	1.7		0.2
Cheerios, 1oz	111	1.8	0.8	0.3		0.4
Cocoa Puffs, 1oz	109	1.0				
Corn Flakes, Kel., 1oz	110	0.1				0.1
Froot Loops, 1oz	111	0.5				0.3
Granola, 1oz	126	4.9	0.7	3.3		0.3
Grape-nuts, 1oz	101	0.1				0.5
Puffed rice, 1oz	57	0.1				0.0
Raisen Bran, 1oz	87	0.5				0.9
Special K, 1oz	111	0.1				0.1
Total, 1oz	100	0.6	0.3	0.1		0.5
Wheat germ, 1oz	108	3.0	1.8	0.5		0.7
Wheaties, 1oz	99	0.5	0.2	0.1	2	0.5

CHEESE & CHEESE PRODUCTS

	K Cal	Total Fat (g)	Poly-Uns. Fat (g)	Sat. Fat (g)	Chol (mg)	Fiber (g)
American spread, 1oz	82	6.0	0.2	3.8	16	0.0
American, 1oz	106	8.9	0.3	5.6	27	0.0
Blue, 1oz	100	8.2	0.2	5.3	21	0.0
Brie, 1oz	105	7.9			28	0.0
Cambembert, 1oz	85	6.9	0.2	4.3	20	0.0
Cheddar, 1oz	114	9.4	0.3	6.0	30	0.0

	K Cal	Total Fat (g)	Poly-Uns. Fat (g)	Sat. Fat (g)	Chol (mg)	Fiber (g)
Cottage, 1% fat 4oz	164	2.3	0.0	1.5	10	0.0
Cottage, creamed 4oz	117	5.1	0.2	3.2	17	0.0
Cream cheese, 1oz	99	9.9	0.4	6.2	31	0.0
Feta, 1oz	75	6.0	0.2	4.2	25	0.0
Mozzarella, 1oz	80	6.1	0.2	3.7	22	0.0
Mozzarella, part skim 1oz	72	4.5	0.1	2.9	16	0.0
Muenster, 1oz	104	8.5	0.2	5.4	27	0.0
Parmesan, 1oz	111	7.3	0.2	4.7	19	0.0
Roquefort, 1oz	105	8.7	0.4	5.5	26	0.0
Swiss, 1oz	96	7.8	0.3	5.0	26	0.0

CHIPS & SNACKS

	K Cal	Total Fat (g)	Poly-Uns. Fat (g)	Sat. Fat (g)	Chol (mg)	Fiber (g)
Bugles, 1oz	150	8.0				
Cheese puffs, 1oz	159	10.0			1	0.1
Corn chips, 1oz	153	8.8				
Cracker jacks, 1oz	114	1.0				
Popcorn, 1cup	54	0.7				0.3
Potato chips, 1oz	153	9.8			0	0.4
Potato frlies, 1oz	158	10.1				0.4
Pretzels	111	1.0				0.1
Tortilla chips, 1oz	139	6.6			0	0.3

EGGS & EGG SUBSTITUTES

	K Cal	Total Fat (g)	Poly-Uns. Fat (g)	Sat. Fat (g)	Chol (mg)	Fiber (g)
Crepe, apple 1crepe	195	5.0			15	
Egg beaters, 1/4cup	30	0.0			0	
Egg white, 1lg	16	0.0	0.0	0.0	0	0.0
Egg yolk, 1lg	63	5.6	0.7	1.7	272	0.0
Egg, fried, 1lg	83	6.4	0.7	2.4	246	0.0
Egg, hard/soft, 1lg	79	5.6	0.7	1.7	274	0.0
Egg, scramb w/milk&fat	95	7.1	0.7	2.8	248	0.0

	K Cal	Total Fat (g)	Poly-Uns. Fat (g)	Sat. Fat (g)	Chol (mg)	Fiber (g)
Omlet, spanish 8oz	250	18.0				
Quiche lorraine, 9.5oz	720	41.0			95	
Souffle, cheese 4oz	240	18.8				

FAST FOODS

ARBY'S
Club sandwich	560	30.0			100	
Roast beef sandwich	350	15.0			45	

ARTHUR TREACHER
Chicken, fried filet	369	21.6	5.6			
Chips	275	13.1	2.7			
Fish, fried	354	19.7	5.6			
Krunch pup(hot dog)	204	14.9	2.2			
Shrimp, fried	381	24.4	6.2			
BURGER CHEF						
Cheeseburger	290	13.0			39	0.2
Cheeseburger, double	420	22.0			77	0.2
French fries, large	351	26.0			0	0.9
Hambaerger, big chef	569	36.0			81	0.3
Hot chocolate	198	8.0			30	
Rancher platter	640	42.0			106	1.3
Shake, choc	403	9.0			36	

BURGER KING
Cheeseburger	350	17.0				
Cheeseburger, double	530	32.0				
Hamburger, whopper	630	36.0				
Onion rings	270	16.0				
Shake, choc	340	10.0				

	K Cal	Total Fat (g)	Poly- Uns. Fat (g)	Sat. Fat (g)	Chol (mg)	Fiber (g)
CHURCH'S FRIED CHICKEN						
Chicken,dark fried 3.5oz	305	21.0				0.2
Chicken,white fried 3.5oz	327	23.0				0.1
DAIRY QUEEN						
Banana split	540	15.0			30	
Float	330	8.0			20	
Freeze	520	13.0			35	
Ice cream cone, med	230	7.0			20	
Shake, med	600	20.0			50	
Sundae, choc, med	290	7.0			20	
LONG JOHN SILVER						
Chicken planks, 4	457	23.0				
Clam chowder	107	3.0				
Fish sandwich	560	31.0				
Oysers, breaded 6	441	19.0				
Shrimp w/batter 6	268	13.0				
MCDONALD'S						
Big mac	563	33.0			86	0.6
Cheeseburger	307	14.1			37	0.2
Chicken mcnugget 6	314	19.0			76	
Egg mcmuffin	327	14.8			229	0.1
English muffin w/butter	186	5.3			13	0.1
French fries, reg	220	11.5			9	0.5
Hash brown potatoes	125	7.0			7	0.3
Quarter pounder	424	21.7			67	0.7
Quarter pounder w/cheese	524	30.7			96	0.8
Sausage, pork	206	18.6			43	0.1